# The Canadian Paramedic: An Introduction

## A Supplement to Mosby's Paramedic Textbook

**Rob Theriault, EMCA, RCT (Adv.), CCP(F)**
Professor, Paramedic Program
Georgian College
Barrie, Ontario

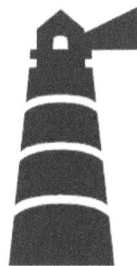

JONES & BARTLETT
LEARNING

*World Headquarters*
Jones & Bartlett Learning
5 Wall Street
Burlington, MA 01803
978-443-5000
info@jblearning.com
www.jblearning.com

Jones & Bartlett Learning books and products are available through most bookstores and online booksellers.
To contact Jones & Bartlett Learning directly, call 800-832-0034, fax 978-443-8000, or visit our website, www.jblearning.com.

Substantial discounts on bulk quantities of Jones & Bartlett Learning publications are available to corporations, professional associations, and other qualified organizations. For details and specific discount information, contact the special sales department at Jones & Bartlett Learning via the above contact information or send an email to specialsales@jblearning.com.

**Production Credits**

Chief Executive Officer: Ty Field
President: James Homer
SVP, Editor-in-Chief: Michael Johnson
SVP, Chief Marketing Officer: Alison M. Pendergast
Executive Publisher: Kimberly Brophy
Executive Acquisitions Editor—EMS: Christine Emerton
Vice President of Sales, Public Safety Group: Matthew Maniscalco
Director of Sales, Public Safety Group: Patricia Einstein

Production Assistant: Kristen Rogers
Director of Marketing: Alisha Weisman
VP, Manufacturing and Inventory Control: Therese Connell
Director of Photo Research and Permissions: Amy Wrynn
Printing and Binding: Courier Companies
Cover Printing: Courier Companies

**To order this product, use ISBN:** 978-1-2840-3805-7

**Library and Archives Canada Cataloguing in Publication**
Theriault, Rob, 1959–
The Canadian paramedic: an introduction: a Canadian supplement to
Mosby's paramedic textbook / Rob Theriault.
Includes index.
ISBN 0-7796-9928-9
1. Emergency medicine—Textbooks. I. Title.
RC86.7.T458 2006 616.02'5 C2006-903588-1

6048

Printed in the United States of America
16 15 14 13 12   10 9 8 7 6 5 4 3 2 1

*To my wife Stacey and daughter Madeline,*
*for their support during the development*
*of this project.*

*To Jim Scribner,*
*former British Columbia Ambulance*
*Service Unit Chief, Whistler,*
*who inspired me to teach.*

# CONTRIBUTORS

**Aileen A. Ashman, RN, LLM**
Barrister and Solicitor
Sharon, Ontario
*Chapter 3: Medical-Legal Aspects of Paramedic Practice*

**Eric Glass, Paramedic**
Chairman
Paramedic Association of Manitoba
Winnipeg, Manitoba
*Chapter 1: Introduction to Paramedic Practice*

**Paul Morneau, BSc, ACP**
Chairman, Government and Media Relations
Paramedic Association of Canada
Ottawa, Ontario
*Chapter 1: Introduction to Paramedic Practice*

**Michael J. Murray, MD, CCFP(EM)**
Chief of Staff
Royal Victoria Hospital
Barrie, Ontario
Medical Director, Base Hospital Program for
    Simcoe/Muskoka
Chair, Ontario Base Hospital Group Medical
    Advisory Committee
*Appendix B—Canadian Triage Acuity Scale*

**Mike Plato, EMT-P**
Superintendent
Emergency Medical Services
The City of Calgary
Calgary, Alberta
*Chapter 1: Introduction to Paramedic Practice*

**Christopher D. Robertson, BA, PG Cert (Ed),
    EMCA, CCP(F)**
Quality and Development Manager (Deputy Chief)
Hastings-Quinte EMS
Belleville, Ontario
*Chapter 1: Introduction to Paramedic Practice*
*Chapter 3: Medical-Legal Aspects of Paramedic Practice*

**Rob Theriault, EMCA, RCT (Adv.), CCP(F)**
Professor, Paramedic Program
Georgian College
Barrie, Ontario
*Chapter 1: Introduction to Paramedic Practice*
*Chapter 2: Injury Prevention and Health Promotion*
*Chapter 3: Medical-Legal Aspects of Paramedic Practice*
*Appendix A—Canadian Emergency Drug Index*

# PREFACE

This supplement is designed to be studied along with the extensive information already in *Mosby's Paramedic Textbook*. It provides information specific to the paramedic profession in Canada.

While the patients we see in the field in Canada are not that different from those in the United States, our countries do differ in many ways. In Canada, we enjoy a universal healthcare system, which means that paramedics do not have to concern themselves with whether the patient has the right insurance or is able to pay for services. Our laws governing health care and paramedic practice are also different. Our education system for paramedics is distinct from that of the United States, and some of the drugs used in the two countries differ.

In Canada, we recently developed the National Occupational Competency Profiles (NOCP), which describe in some detail three levels of paramedic practice. We also recently made the very important decision to apply the title of *paramedic* to all entry level professional ambulance personnel who are authorized to perform controlled medical acts. This landmark decision will solidify our identity as a unified profession.

*The Canadian Paramedic: An Introduction* contains three chapters and three appendices designed to address aspects of paramedic practice that are distinctly Canadian. **Chapter 1: Introduction to Paramedic Practice** discusses EMS history in Canada, EMS systems, education, levels of care, paramedic subspecialties, and professionalism. **Chapter 2: Injury Prevention and Health Promotion** covers the primary causes of injury and injury-related deaths in Canada, effective strategies for reducing injuries, and the role of paramedics in this important field. The paramedic's role in health promotion is also discussed.

**Chapter 3: Medical–Legal Aspects of Paramedic Practice** includes an overview of the legal system in Canada, a discussion of specific laws governing paramedic practice, and simple steps that must be taken to avoid legal liability.

**Appendix A: Canadian Emergency Drug Index (EDI)** contains a listing of 12 drugs used in Canada and not included in the EDI of the main textbook. **Appendix B: Canadian Triage Acuity Scale** describes the new triage system that is currently employed in hospital emergency departments across Canada and is rapidly making its way into EMS systems. **Appendix C: National Occupational Competency Profiles** defines and describes the National Occupational Competency Profiles and connects them to key chapters in the textbook and supplement.

As in *Mosby's Paramedic Textbook,* each chapter begins with a list of objectives that provide an overview of the material to be presented. This allows the student to review the content and progression of each chapter in an easy-to-follow format. The objectives are followed by an alphabetical listing of key terms found in the chapter. This is complemented by a glossary of terms in the back of the book. Because the Canadian and American systems are distinct, we have made changes, where appropriate, to several key terms that are also found in the glossary of the main text. This is particularly important as it applies to medical–legal terminology.

I hope that you find the information in this supplement helpful, whether you are an educator, student, working paramedic, or ambulance service operator. I look forward to your feedback so that we can continue to strive to meet the needs of all Canadian paramedic students.

Rob Theriault
rtheriault@georgianc.on.ca

# ACKNOWLEDGMENTS

I would like to thank the following people:

My editor, Toni Chahley, whose guidance, constant encouragement, and attention to detail have helped me grow as a writer and in coordinating the efforts of several contributing authors for this, my first published book;

All the reviewers, whose experiences, insights, and thoughtful comments have helped make this a better supplement;

Andrew Robert, Director of the County of Simcoe Paramedic Service, whose experience and wisdom helped me better appreciate the challenges of ambulance service operations and the qualities that make a paramedic a great asset to the service and to the community;

Jocelyn Bourgoin, Director of Superior EMS, who has always been a great source of information about the challenges of paramedic practice and volunteerism in rural and remote Canada.

# REVIEWERS

**Mary-Ann Clarkes, EMT**
Director of Administration
Canadian College of Emergency Medical Services
Edmonton, Alberta

**Robert Conn, MD FRCSC**
President & CEO
SMARTRISK
Toronto, Ontario

**Craig Desjardins, EMCA, ACP**
ACP/PCP Coordinator
Atlantic Paramedic Academy/Academie paramedicale
    de l'Atlantique
Moncton, NB

**Sean Fisher, PCP**
Fire & Paramedic Instructor, Manitoba Emergency
Services College
Brandon, Manitoba

**Cameron Glass, EMT-P**
Coordinator, Advanced Care Programs
Justice Institute of British Columbia Paramedic Academy
New Westminster, British Columbia

**René Lapierre, A-EMCA, ACP**
Professor, Paramedic Program, Collège Boréal
Advance Care Paramedic ACP/PCP Preceptor
Sudbury, Ontario

**Martin McNamara, MD CCFP (EM)**
Assistant Clinical Professor, McMaster University
Hamilton, Ontario
President, Medical Staff, Huronia District Hospital
Midland, Ontario
Medical Director, Paramedic Program, Humber College
Toronto, Ontario

# CONTENTS

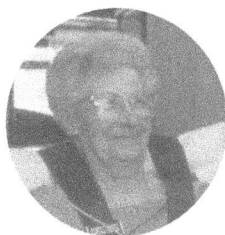

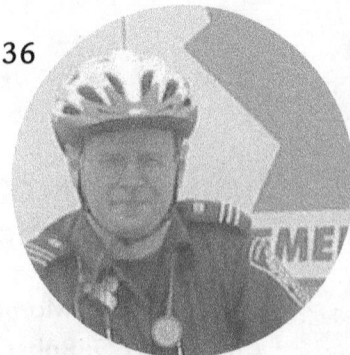

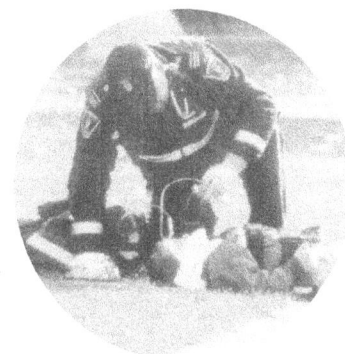

# CHAPTER

# 1 Introduction to Paramedic Practice

## ● ● ● OBJECTIVES

*Upon completion of this chapter, the paramedic student will be able to:*

1. Outline key historical events that influenced the development of emergency medical services (EMS) systems in Canada.
2. Identify the key elements necessary for effective EMS systems operations.
3. Differentiate the training and roles and responsibilities of the three nationally recognized levels of paramedic licensure/certification: Primary Care, Advanced Care, and Critical Care Paramedic.
4. List the benefits of membership in professional paramedic organizations.
5. Describe the benefits of continuing medical education.

6. Differentiate between professionalism and professional licensure, certification, and registration.
7. Identify the responsibilities and accountabilities required of a professional.
8. Describe and distinguish offline (indirect) from online (direct) medical direction.
9. Define and explain the concept of medical directives.
10. List and justify the rationale for various paramedic subspecialties.
11. Explain the components and the role of an effective total quality management program.

## ● ● ● KEY TERMS

Advanced Care Paramedic (ACP) ... 11
advanced life support (ALS) ... 3
attending or lead paramedic ... 7
automated external defibrillator (AED) ... 6
automatic vehicle location (AVL) ... 6
basic life support (BLS) ... 3
continuous quality improvement (CQI) ... 20
controlled medical act ... 3
Critical Care Paramedic (CCP) ... 11
cultural competence ... 13
differential diagnosis ... 6
emergency medical services (EMS) ... 3
emergency medical technician (EMT) ... 3
first responder ... 6
hemodynamic monitoring device ... 11
history of the presenting illness/injury (HPI) ... 6

hospital diversion ... 7
incident management system (IMS) ... 16
mass casualty incident (MCI) ... 6
mechanical ventilator ... 11
medical directive ... 7
out-of-hospital care ... 4
prehospital ... 2
Primary Care Paramedic (PCP) ... 10
primary problem ... 6
provisional diagnosis or field diagnosis ... 6
reciprocity ... 12
scope of practice ... 11
standing order ... 10
total quality management (TQM) ... 19
triage bypass ... 7
triage nurse ... 7

This Canadian supplement and *Mosby's Paramedic Textbook* are designed to meet the needs of both the layperson who is entering the paramedic field and the working paramedic who has chosen to advance his or her career.

If you are just entering this field as a Primary Care Paramedic, you are about to embark on a unique career path with exciting challenges. Your work environment, unlike the clinical setting where many other healthcare professionals work, is chaotic and sometimes harsh by nature—both metaphorically and literally. Your expertise as a paramedic will reflect your knowledge, decision-making ability, professional demeanour, and patient care skills. You also need the capacity to adjust your treatment plans swiftly and seamlessly in the face of the patient's rapidly changing medical condition and within a wide range of environmental conditions. Every paramedic call is different, and the environment can change dramatically from one call to the next. One moment you may be treating a patient having a seizure in the middle of a crowded shopping mall, and the next hour you may be drawing up life-saving drugs in the dark of night at the base of a steep cliff in subzero temperatures.

The rewards for your efforts will rarely come directly from grateful patients or their families. Instead they will come from the knowledge that you were a calming influence in their time of crisis and that your decision-making abilities and skilled hands helped bring about a positive outcome. If you have chosen this path because you genuinely want to help people, the care and kindness you provide will serve as its own reward and will carry you through an entire career with a sense of purpose and pride.

If you are a paramedic who plans to pursue Advanced Care Paramedic (ACP) certification, your new role will encompass a scope of practice and level of responsibility that will enrich your career even further. You will acquire a deeper knowledge and understanding of clinical field practice, learn new life-saving and life-impacting skills, and reap the rewards that come with challenging yourself and providing a higher level of care.

## HISTORY OF THE EMERGENCY MEDICAL SERVICES SYSTEM

### Before the Twentieth Century

Paramedicine has its roots in the transportation of the sick and the injured. **Prehospital** care originated primarily with the military through the ages and the need to safely move injured soldiers from the battlefield to a hospital. In A.D. 900, the first wagon for transporting invalids was constructed by the Anglo-Saxons.[1] One hundred and sixty years later, the Normans introduced the design of a horse litter, which remained a standard of transportation, with variations of the original design, until the seventeenth century.[1] However, it was not until the early 1790s that ambulances were conceived in France by Dr. Dominique-John Larrey, Chief of Surgery to Napoleon's Imperial Guard.[2] They were designed primarily to transport medical personnel to the site of an injured person, rather than transporting the injured from the site to a hospital. Ambulances were, in fact, known as *field hospitals,* from the French term "hôpital ambulant," or moving hospital. In 1792, Dr. Larrey introduced the first ambulances staffed with medically trained personnel who carried the wounded from the battlefield to a hospital. This proved to be a safer and more efficient means of treating injured soldiers.[2]

In Canada, the earliest known ambulance was a horse-drawn wagon donated to the Toronto General Hospital by an anonymous female benefactor in 1880.[2] In the late nineteenth and early twentieth centuries, since it was not always possible for the sick to make their way to a doctor, ambulances served to transport physicians to the bedside and, only when necessary, to transport patients to the hospital.

### Beyond the Twentieth Century

In 1905, Major Pallister of the Canadian militia made an interesting contribution to the military ambulance with the design of an armoured three-wheeled vehicle bearing the symbol of the Red Cross.[1] It appears to be the first motorized ambulance in Canada and had an 18-horsepower gasoline motor. It travelled at an astounding 10 km an hour over rough terrain. In 1912, Connelly-McKinley Funeral Homes, in Edmonton, Alberta, introduced what was probably the first motorized civilian ambulance in Canada.[3] The second motorized civilian ambulance in Canada was purchased at the request of Dr. N.A. Pownell, Senior Assistant Surgeon at the Toronto General Hospital, in May, 1913.[2]

From the early part of the 1900s until the 1970s, Canadian civilian ambulance services were run largely by funeral homes as a sideline. During this time, with few exceptions, ambulances functioned essentially as "taxis for the horizontal."[2] Staff were referred to as ambulance drivers, since the only requirements for employment in most cases were basic first aid and a chauffeur's licence.

Despite the technological advances in the transportation industry and the improving speed and comfort of ambulances in the ensuing years, medical care on ambulances was slower to progress. The responsibility for ambulance services and the role of ambulance personnel remained unclear through the first two thirds of the twentieth century. Ambulance personnel worked for funeral homes, hospitals, police departments, fire services, and privately run ambulance services. No single organization was willing to make a commitment to those who chose ambulance work and proudly called it their profession. Ambulance personnel were, in essence, foster children, spending some of their time with the healthcare family and at other times bounced between emergency services families.

Wartime evidence in support of medical interventions at the scene was slow to make its way into civilian prehospital care but would eventually help define the role of ambulance personnel. As this evolution unfolded, the continuing lack of clear direction was due largely to an ongoing debate over the role of the ambulance: Was it merely to transport the sick or the injured to the hospital? Or was it to take skilled healthcare professionals to the scene, where medical interventions could be initiated and continued en route to a hospital?

Over the period of the World Wars, the Korean War, and the Vietnam War, mortality among soldiers injured on the battlefield declined from 8% to less than 2% due to improvements in front-line prehospital care and increasing sophistication and speed of transportation.[4] The knowledge gained from these conflicts would serve as a catalyst to the evolution of civilian ambulance systems, raising them from disorganized systems of transportation to today's sophisticated prehospital care and transportation systems.

## EMERGENCY MEDICAL SERVICES SYSTEMS TODAY

Modern **emergency medical services (EMS)** systems owe their origins to the military experience. The word "paramedic" is derived from *para* meaning "beside" and *medic* meaning "medical." In the battlefield, though, paramedics did not always work alongside physicians. They received training and medical orders from physicians, as they do today, and acted as the eyes, ears, and hands of the physician on the front lines, performing life-saving procedures.

In the postwar era, Canada's EMS systems began to blossom. Canadians looked to the U.S. model of organized systems and the different levels of **emergency medical technician (EMT)** training. In Ontario, in 1966, Dr. Norman H. McNally was hired by the Ontario provincial government to create an integrated ambulance service. Dr. McNally is credited with formalizing education for ambulance personnel, first with the development of the Fundamentals of Casualty Care Program out of Canadian Forces Base Borden, and later with the establishment of ambulance and emergency care programs at community colleges across the province in 1975.[2] In 1974, the government of British Columbia addressed the concerns over various ambulance operators and varying standards of care by enacting legislation to create the British Columbia Ambulance Service (BCAS).[5]

In the 1960s and 1970s, EMS systems and paramedicine as a profession in Canada were in their infancy.

Community colleges and other educational institutions began training select ambulance personnel to perform medical interventions such as drug administration and other **advanced life support (ALS)** interventions. ALS, at that time, was synonymous with "paramedic." This was an exciting beginning, but it also created confusion for the public: Would they receive advanced life support from a paramedic or **basic life support (BLS)** from an ambulance attendant?

Despite postwar evidence in support of advanced training for prehospital personnel, debates continued: Are paramedics healthcare professionals, emergency services personnel, or both? What is the optimum service model for prehospital care? Is it hospital based? Independent? Connected to a fire department? How much training should ambulance personnel receive? Should they all be trained to the ALS level? Should they all be trained to a BLS level only? Or should there be a mix of BLS and ALS providers? How much time should be spent on the scene? What medical interventions should be performed on the scene? What interventions should be postponed until the patient is en route to the hospital? What interventions should be postponed until they can be performed by a doctor at the hospital?

These ongoing discussions were part of the excitement as EMS systems took shape. They also reflected the identity crisis of a profession growing up and trying to establish itself as a unique and valuable contributor to society.

In the latter half of the twentieth century, the term *paramedic* was more broadly defined to include all qualified ambulance personnel who are certified to perform one or more **controlled medical acts**.

Paramedic training has expanded dramatically in Canada. Today most ambulances, with the exception of many in rural and remote regions, are staffed with qualified paramedics. Paramedics are no longer in the exclusive business of transporting the ill or the injured to the hospital (see Paramedic Subspecialties). They provide sophisticated emergency medical care on the scene, in a variety of settings, and, if transport is indicated, en route to the hospital.

In keeping with the tenets of healthcare professions, the care provided by paramedics is coming under increasing scientific scrutiny. This is a positive advancement for the profession and means that prehospital research will help ensure that the care paramedics provide is supported by medical evidence. Organizations such as the Canadian EHS Research Consortium (http://cerc.paramedic.ca/) are helping to promote and facilitate out-of-hospital research and to educate paramedics about research.

Paramedicine has entered an exciting and turbulent period of adolescence. Through this phase, our growth continues rapidly, as we seek our own unique identity within the greater healthcare community and in our relationship with other emergency services such as Fire and Police. As part of this growth, we struggle for a clear and singular identity. Terms such as EMS, ambulance services, and paramedic are found everywhere in Canadian prehos-

**Table 1–1**    Summary of Paramedic Designations, Canadian Medical Association, April 2006

| PROVINCE | PARAMEDIC DESIGNATIONS |
|---|---|
| Alberta | Emergency Medical Responder (EMR)<br>Emergency Medical Technician (EMT)<br>Emergency Medical Technologist–Paramedic (EMT-P) |
| British Columbia | EMAFR<br>EMR<br>Primary Care Paramedic (PCP)<br>Advanced Care Paramedic (ACP)<br>Critical Care Paramedic (CCP)<br>Infant Transport Team (ITT) Paramedic |
| Manitoba | First Responder<br>EMA I<br>EMA II<br>EMA III |
| New Brunswick<br>Newfoundland and Labrador | EMT-I<br>EMR I<br>EMR II<br>Paramedic 1<br>Paramedic 2<br>PCP |
| Nova Scotia | PCP (P1)<br>ICP (Intermediate Care Paramedic)<br>ACP (P3)<br>CCP |
| Ontario | Advanced Emergency Medical Care Attendant (AEMCA) (entry-to-practice credential)<br>PCP (minimum requirement for employment)<br>ACP (provincial certification before title can be used)<br>CCP |
| Prince Edward Island | EMT-I (P-1/PCP)<br>EMT-II (P-2)<br>EMT-III (P-3/ACP) |
| Quebec | First Responder<br>Ambulance Technician<br>Ambulance Technician in Advanced Prehospital Setting |
| Saskatchewan | First Responder<br>EMR<br>EMT<br>EMT-A<br>EMT-P |

Note: Designations were not available for the territories.

pital care. To people in the industry, the terms are clear; however, imagine the confusion for the layperson when a passing ambulance has lettering reading Ambulance, EMS, and Paramedics.

Although most ambulances in Canada are staffed with paramedics, the term "paramedic" is not yet used by the lay public universally in this country (see Table 1-1). The evolution of **out-of-hospital care** has helped create and perpetuate this confusion. Over the years, and in particular since 1970, the titles for Canadian ambulance personnel have

changed frequently. Personnel who provide prehospital care have been called, among other terms, ambulance drivers/attendants, ambulance officers, emergency medical attendants/assistants (EMA), EMA I, EMA II, EMA III, emergency medical technicians (EMT), EMT–paramedics, paramedics I, and paramedics II.

In 2001, the Paramedic Association of Canada (PAC) established national occupational competency profiles for three paramedic levels. Paramedicine has since become the acceptable entry level to practice.

Now that paramedic care is increasingly becoming the standard in out-of-hospital care, does it still make sense to define paramedic services by the ambulances in which many, but not all, paramedics work? Paramedics work in many other settings: boats, temporary or permanent structures at mass gatherings, helicopters, airplanes, and even hospitals.

Paramedics should no more be identified with the vehicle in which many of them work than a police constable would be identified with a police car or a firefighter with a fire truck. Paramedics are not in the transportation business. They are in the business of patient care; transportation is a supporting role. They provide much more than a ride to the hospital.

*Emergency medical services* is another term that once served an important purpose in broadly describing a system in which paramedics and others worked. It has also been broadly used to encompass anyone, including the lay public and other emergency services personnel, who plays a role in prehospital care.

Since *paramedic* is fast becoming the single standard term in Canada to define out-of-hospital professionals, do terms such as *EMS* and *ambulance* only add confusion? Will they one day become obsolete? These questions can only be answered with time, further debate, and consensus.

## EMS Symbols

In 1864, the first Geneva Convention, signed in Geneva, Switzerland, by the leaders of 12 countries, spelled out the first internationally accepted rules for the humane treatment of wounded soldiers. About the same time, international relief committees were formed that grew into the Red Cross organization. The red cross emerged as a sign identifying vehicles, hospitals, and personnel who cared for injured soldiers. The red cross, and later the red crescent, became symbols of a place of refuge for the injured in countries throughout the world.[2]

Until the 1970s, the red cross was widely used to represent both military and civilian EMS systems. However, a later Geneva Convention restricted its use to the International Red Cross organization alone. The blue star of life (see Figure 1–1) replaced the red cross as a symbol representing EMS. Created in 1973 by Leo R. Schwartz, Chief of the EMS Branch of the U.S. National Highway Traffic Safety Administration (NHTSA), it consists of a six-pointed star with the Rod of Asclepius in the centre. The star of life was registered in 1977 and recognized by the American Medical Association as the symbol that would identify EMS organizations and certified personnel.

The six branches of the star are symbols of the six main tasks executed by rescuers all through the emergency chain:

1. The first rescuers, often lay people, arrive on the scene, observe the scene, understand the problem, identify the dangers to themselves and the patient(s), and take appropriate measures to ensure safety at the scene.
2. The first rescuers call for professional help.
3. The first rescuers provide first aid and immediate care to the extent of their capabilities.
4. The EMS personnel arrive and provide immediate care to the extent of their capabilities.
5. The EMS personnel transfer the patient to a hospital for specialized care. They provide medical care during the transportation.
6. Appropriate specialized care is provided at the hospital.

One can see how the system has changed since the creation of the star of life. Although it continues to be an important symbol of who we are and the work that we do, perhaps it is time to modify the descriptions of the six tasks. For instance, in task 5, the vague term "EMS personnel" should be replaced with the term "paramedic" to give greater clarity to the public and promote universality of the paramedic profession. And tasks 5 and 6 could be modified to acknowledge that some patients receive specialized care in the field and do not require transportation.

## EMS Operations

Paramedics bring medical expertise and patient care to the community in times of acute illness or injury. They are part of a larger community of caregivers and services that include the lay public, 911, emergency medical dispatchers (EMD), medical directors, firefighters and police, community healthcare professionals, hospitals, and rehabilitation specialists. Smooth coordination among all these providers and services forms the chain of survival. Each link in the chain is interdependent with the other. Each provides a unique contribution. Paramedics must work to support and promote all links in the best interests of the patient.

### THE ROLE OF THE PUBLIC

When an emergency happens, the public expects a rapid response and a high level of medical care. From taxpayers

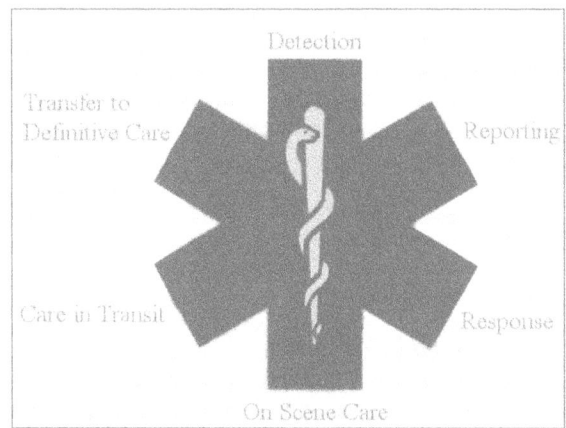

FIGURE 1–1 The star of life.

in a universal healthcare system, this is a reasonable expectation. However, receiving medical attention outside of the hospital environment is not necessarily as intuitive as one might think. First, it requires that someone, either the patient or a bystander, recognizes that a medical emergency exists. Next, it requires someone to activate the system so that paramedics, and other emergency services if required, respond. Case in point: The vast majority of patients experiencing a heart attack will take three hours or more to make the decision to seek medical attention.[6] To address this problem, paramedics, cardiopulmonary resuscitation (CPR) instructors and the medical community have worked hard for years to educate the lay public to recognize the signs and symptoms of a heart attack and call 911 quickly. While some communities have had some success in educating the lay public, many more have had minimal impact.[6]

On a positive note, public training in CPR has lowered mortality for cardiac arrest: an important potential saving of lives, since there are between 35,000 and 45,000 cases of cardiac arrest in Canada each year.[7] The teaching of CPR and the use of public access defibrillation (PAD) by the lay public for potential victims of sudden death has resulted in survival rates as high as 74% where **automated external defibrillators (AED)** are made available in public places.[8] The key to success is that anyone can be trained to use these machines safely, and people already on the scene can respond more quickly to victims of cardiac arrest than can paramedics or other emergency service personnel.

Imagine another scene, for example, involving a pedestrian struck by a car at a busy intersection. Several people are there who witnessed the incident, yet it takes longer than one might expect for paramedics to arrive on the scene. It turns out that while there were several witnesses, most assumed that a person close to the incident holding a cell phone was talking to the 911 dispatcher, when in fact she was talking to a friend. People assumed that someone else had called 911, yet no one did until many minutes had passed.

Thus, the chain of survival depends on the public recognizing that an emergency exists, taking the next step of calling 911 or the local emergency number to activate the system, and, in the best-case scenario, providing basic first aid or CPR to the best of their abilities until paramedics arrive. Paramedics, as the experts in prehospital care, are ideally suited to educate the public in first aid, CPR, and PAD, and to speak to matters of health promotion, injury prevention (see Chapter 2), and when to call 911 for medical emergencies.

## MAKING THE 911 CALL

When an acute illness or injury strikes, a citizen calls 911. The 911 dispatcher will inquire whether this is a call for police, fire, or ambulance. The 911 dispatcher then, in the case of a medical emergency, transfers the call to an emergency medical dispatcher (EMD). EMDs are usually the first point of communication with the patient or a bystander. They are the essential link between the acutely ill or the injured and life-saving medical care. Their role is to first confirm the location of the call, then calmly determine the nature and priority of the emergency and allocate all appropriate resources. This may mean a paramedic response, fire and paramedic response, or, in the event of a **mass casualty incident (MCI)**, all necessary emergency services, including police and allied agencies, such as the air ambulance, hydro, the coroner, or neighbouring emergency services. Many EMD centres have technologies such as **automatic vehicle location (AVL)** and global positioning systems (GPS) to help the dispatcher locate the closest ambulance and direct it to the call scene if necessary.

EMDs frequently handle multiple calls simultaneously and coordinate ambulance transport with the closest and most appropriate hospital. In addition, while one EMD is dispatching a paramedic crew, another will stay on the line with the caller while the paramedics are on their way, to provide first-aid or CPR instructions, instruct a father or friend in the delivery of a baby, or talk a patient out of committing suicide. This requires an individual with exceptional communication and problem-solving skills and the ability to multitask and to work quickly under tremendous pressure. EMDs are often instrumental in saving lives and rarely receive the recognition they deserve.

## PREHOSPITAL CARE

Within seconds of the call being received by the EMD, the closest or most appropriate paramedic crew is sent to the scene while the dispatcher obtains further details from the caller. A crew of PCPs or ACPs or of both may be dispatched, depending on the information. In some urban areas, Critical Care Paramedics (CCPs) may also be used. In a number of remote areas, the only available responders may be emergency medical responders (EMRs) or **first responders**.

Regardless of your level of certification, your role as the crew on the scene is to manage the scene and care for the patient or patients to the best of your abilities and within your scope of practice. This involves first determining whether the scene is safe (e.g., from fallen electrical wires, fire, potential violence, toxic spills). Next, you have to uncover and begin to correct any life-threatening conditions that affect the airway, breathing, or circulation (ABCs). The rest of your examination consists of ascertaining the patient's chief complaint, eliciting a **history of the presenting illness or injury (HPI)**, past medical history, medications, and allergies, taking vital signs, using other diagnostic tools as necessary, and conducting a head-to-toe examination. During the process of the examination, you will be formulating a **differential diagnosis**, or a short list of possible causes of the patient's complaint. Finally, you will establish a **provisional diagnosis** (sometimes referred to as a *field diagnosis*), which is the most likely cause of the presenting signs and symptoms or the **primary problem**. Unlike physicians, paramedics do not "diagnose" illness or injury in the true sense of the term. However, in order to initiate treatment, you will need to narrow the list of possible causes to one for which your treatment plan is safe and beneficial to the patient. For example, suppose you encounter a patient who is having difficulty breathing, has a history of asthma and an allergy to cats, and is visiting a friend who owns a cat. If, when you listen to the patient's chest with your stethoscope, you hear wheezing, and if all other assessment findings point in the same direction, your provisional diagnosis will be an acute exacerbation of asthma.

Your greatest asset as a paramedic is your ability to perform a focused and rapid assessment. Your knowledge and experience will form the foundation of an accurate assessment. Without these foundational elements, the technical skills of performing medical procedures and administering medication are meaningless and potentially dangerous. Your knowledge and decision-making skills are critical for weighing the benefit-to-risk ratio of all medical interventions.

Not all "prehospital" care results in transportation of a patient to the hospital. In some cases, paramedics are able to provide sufficient and appropriate care at the scene to enable the patient to recover and then remain at home and care for himself or herself. For example, one of the more common medical emergencies paramedics respond to is a diabetic with low blood sugar. In some instances, you may be able to render treatment, correct the blood sugar, and leave the patient with another caregiver, such as a family member, who can provide food and supervision.

In most cases, however, you will be assessing, treating, and transporting patients to the hospital. A series of events must occur for a smooth transfer of care from the prehospital to the in-hospital setting.

## HOSPITAL CARE

On most calls that you respond to as a paramedic, you will transport the patient(s) to the closest hospital. In the rural setting, there may only be one hospital, which makes the destination decision easy. In fact, given Canada's size and the concentration of healthcare facilities in urban areas, you may be required to transport patients for 3–6 hours from the scene to the closest hospital if you work far from a major city. Paramedics working in rural and remote areas may be the most highly trained healthcare professionals in the area. They also have a great deal more to consider with respect to anticipating and preparing for changes in the patient's condition. They must ensure that there are enough medical supplies on board the ambulance for the long transportation.

Paramedics working in an urban setting will sometimes be faced with emergency room (ER) overcrowding and may be asked by the EMD to bypass the closest hospital to go to a less busy one. In some centres, hospitals refer to this as being on "**hospital diversion,**" or on "consideration," meaning they are too busy to take any patients other than those with an immediate life-threatening condition. The

term "**triage bypass**" is used to describe a protocol that allows paramedics to bypass a closer hospital to transport a patient to one with specialized care. Some regions have instituted bypass protocols. A local **medical directive**, applying strict diagnostic and clinical criteria, might allow paramedics to bypass the closest hospital to transport certain patients to a more appropriate hospital where they can receive the best possible care. For example, not all hospitals will have a neurosurgeon on staff for the management of stroke or head injury or an interventional cardiologist on staff to perform procedures such as percutaneous transluminal coronary angioplasty (PTCA).

Once the paramedics arrive at the hospital and the patient is unloaded from the ambulance and brought into the ER, the **attending or lead paramedic** will give a brief patient report to the **triage nurse**. The role of the triage nurse is to sort out all patients, including those in the waiting room, according to priority (see the Canadian Triage Acuity Scale in Appendix B). Once a report on the patient's condition is given to the triage nurse, the patient is assigned a bed. The transfer of care is complete when the paramedics transfer the patient to a hospital bed. There, the attending paramedic is usually expected to give another, more detailed report to the receiving nurse or attending physician.

In the hospital, the patient will likely receive care and services from several healthcare providers, including nurses, physicians, a physician specialist, pharmacists, nutritionists, crisis workers, laboratory personnel, radiology personnel, diagnostic services, and various support staff. In all, an impressive team of experts helps care for patients as they recover from their illness or injury.

## REHABILITATION

After the patient has received a sufficient amount of care and has reached a certain level of independence, the rehabilitation process will begin, if needed. Rehabilitation may begin during or after hospitalization. The services may come in the form of exercise to improve mobility, flexibility, and strength. Some patients may require social services to help them reintegrate into society and the workforce, while others may require new job training that allows them to adapt to a disability.

From the time of illness or injury to the time of recovery and reintegration into the community, the strength of each step is critical to allow patients to return to their optimal potential. Paramedics play a vital link in that chain of survival, recovery, and return to a productive life.

## Types of EMS Delivery Models

Over the past century, Canada has seen many out-of-hospital care delivery models. The best model of service delivery is still being debated. Since the advent of organized EMS systems, the diversity of service providers has narrowed. Today, the vast majority of organized EMS systems are operated directly by municipalities or subcontracted to hospitals or private operators.

## PROVINCIAL OR TERRITORIAL SERVICES

The provinces and territories regulate and fund ambulance services in Canada. However, with the exception of the British Columbia Ambulance Service, some services run by the First Nations, and a few services operated by regions, most services are operated at the municipal level, contracted to a private provider, or operated by the local hospital.

## UPPER-TIER MUNICIPALITY SERVICES

In many provinces and territories, the delivery of ambulance services is municipal based. Many regions and cities across Canada operate their own ambulance services. In most cases, the funding for the services is shared between the province or territory and the upper-tier municipality. This requires a solid municipal tax base, and, as one might imagine, the tax base differs from one municipality to the next and from urban to rural communities. Some rural services lack sufficient funding to recruit and retain paramedics.

## FIRE-BASED EMS SERVICES
## OR EMS-BASED FIRE SERVICES

In contrast with service delivery models in the United States, very few EMS systems in Canada are merged with fire departments. There may be some merit to this concept in smaller communities where the fire call volume is considerably lower than that of the local paramedic service and the sharing of physical space and resources may be beneficial. Another argument in favour of merging operations is the overlap (though small) in calls responded to by both services.

## HOSPITAL-BASED SERVICES

Although hospital-based paramedic systems are less common than in the early twentieth century, even today, several operate in Canada. One of the advantages of a hospital-based system is that paramedics can work closely with physicians and nurses in the emergency department. This type of system may allow for better feedback, allowing paramedics to follow up on the patient's diagnosis and care in the hospital. The close interaction between paramedics and emergency-room staff is also beneficial for ongoing medical education.

## PRIVATE OPERATORS

Some provinces, territories, and municipalities may choose to subcontract ambulance services to a private operator. Private operators may be partially or fully funded by the province, territory, or municipality. For example, the Nova Scotia Department of Health regulates an ambulance service that is managed for the province by a single private

company. Regardless of the funding mechanism, private operators, as with any ambulance operators, are regulated by provincial or territorial legislation (see Table 1–2).

## VOLUNTEER SERVICES

Rural and remote communities across Canada have great difficulty funding ambulance services and recruiting qualified paramedics. Many new graduates are eager to ply their trade in a high-call volume area to gain experience. Remote areas find it difficult to attract paramedics from urban and suburban areas because of a lack of financial incentives and lower call volume, and those who are recruited may leave for better pay or may have difficulty adjusting to a rural lifestyle. Local residents, who would make ideal candidates and who are the main sources of a network of volunteers in the rural setting, frequently lack the means to pursue the necessary education to become qualified paramedics.

Canadians living in these communities have rightly argued that they should have access to an equal level of care. The Romanow Report[9] supports that assertion with the following recommendations:

> **Recommendation 15:**
> A portion of the proposed Rural and Remote Access Fund, the Diagnostic Services Fund, the Primary Health Care Transfer, and the Home Care Transfer should be used to improve the supply and distribution of healthcare providers, encourage changes to their scopes and patterns of practice, and ensure that the best use is made of the mix of skills of different healthcare providers.
> **Recommendation 16:**
> The Health Council of Canada should systematically collect, analyze and regularly report on relevant and necessary information about the Canadian healthcare workforce, including critical issues related to the recruitment, distribution, and remuneration of healthcare providers.
> **Recommendation 30:**
> The Rural and Remote Access Fund should be used to attract and retain healthcare providers.

Addressing the rural and remote staffing issue is a national concern. Paramedic involvement in this issue is critical to helping the public understand the role of paramedics, the level of care they provide, and the need for an equal standard of care for all of the citizens of Canada.

## Medical Direction for Paramedics

With a few jurisdictional exceptions, paramedics are authorized to perform controlled acts only under the authority of a medical director, and only while on duty. Barring local policies to the contrary, performing controlled acts while off duty is not permitted and may, in fact, be grounds for legal action (see Chapter 3).

The medical director may serve the following functions:
- Establish current scopes of practice for paramedics.
- Establish evidence-based medical directives.

**TABLE 1–2** Summary of Provincial Regulations/Legislation Relevant to Paramedics

| PROVINCE | LEGISLATION/REGULATION FOR SCOPE OF PRACTICE | WHO REGULATES? |
|---|---|---|
| Alberta | • *Health Disciplines Act H-2 RSA 2000*<br>• *Emergency Medical Technicians Regulation AR 48/1993*<br>• *Health Professions Act H-7 RSA 2000* | • Ministry of Health and Wellness<br>• Alberta College of Paramedics<br>Registration examinations in place for all levels, including both written and practical evaluations. |
| British Columbia | **Scope of practice is legislated**<br>• *Health Emergency Act (HEA) RSBC 1996 Ch 182 (1974)*<br>• *Emergency Medical Assistants Regulation 562/2004* (Effective January 1, 2005) | • Emergency Medical Assistants Licensing Board<br>Registration examinations in place for all levels |
| Manitoba | • *Ambulance Services Act, CCSM c A65*<br>• *Ambulance Services and Licences Regulation, Man. Reg.133/96* | • Manitoba Health, Emergency Services<br>Registration examinations in place |
| New Brunswick | **Scope of practice not legislated**<br>• *Ambulance Services Act* | • Department of Health and Wellness (via Paramedic Association of New Brunswick) |
| Newfoundland and Labrador | **Scope of practice not legislated**<br>• *Health and Community Services Act SNL 1995 Ch P-37.1* | • Department of Health and Community Services, Board Services |
| Nova Scotia | **Scope of practice not legislated**<br>Scopes of practice are described provincially (EHS Essential Competencies) | • Department of Health, Emergency Health Services (EHS)<br>ACP registration examination in place for paramedics who graduated from an educational program outside Canada |
| Ontario | • *Ambulance Act, RSO 1990, c.A19 and its regulations, O. Reg 257/00* | • Ontario Ministry of Health and Long Term Care, Emergency Health Services Branch<br>Provincial certification for entry-to-practice and Advanced Care Paramedic examinations in place<br>Medical director of base hospital certifies and delegates to paramedics for delivery of controlled medical acts. |
| Prince Edward Island | **Scope of practice is legislated**<br>• *Public Health Act, Part II, Emergency Medical Services*<br>• *Emergency Medical Services Regulations RSPEI 1988, Cap.P-30* | • PEI Department of Health and Social Services, Regulatory Services Division (to become Department of Health, Population Health Division) |
| Quebec | **Scope of practice is legislated**<br>• *An Act respecting pre-hospital emergency services RSQ chapter S-6.2*<br>• *Bylaw on professional activities that can be done in the Emergency Prehospital Services setting, Decree 233-2003, 26 February 2003 law of professions (LRQ, c C-26, 2002, c33* | • Quebec Health and Social Services |
| Saskatchewan | **Scope of practice is not legislated**<br>Scope of practice is described provincially (Saskatchewan Health Scope of Practice Guidelines) | • Saskatchewan Health, Acute and Emergency Services Branch<br>No registration examinations |

Note: Information not available for the territories.
Source: Canadian Medical Association, April 2006.

▓ Ascribe benchmarks for paramedic performance through quality assurance programs in collaboration with the ambulance service provider.

▓ Communicate to paramedics, the Ministry of Health, regional governments, and the public in general, the standards of practice for all levels of paramedics.

▓ Assist in the development and delivery of continuing medical education.

▓ Delineate the medical director's responsibilities and accountabilities.

## ONLINE MEDICAL DIRECTION

Online medical direction refers to direct communication between the medical director or a designated physician and the paramedic in the field. Online medical direction has the unique advantage of linking the medical expertise of the physician with the paramedic. Acting as the "eyes, ears, and hands of the physician," the paramedic is able to convey essential assessment findings to the physician and in turn receive appropriate direction, medical orders, or advice. The physician must have absolute confidence in the paramedic's assessment and description of the patient's condition in order to give orders that are safe and beneficial.

A disadvantage of online medical direction is that communications are not 100% reliable; this can create potential problems when the patient needs any treatment that the paramedic is not authorized to perform without a direct order. Since most medical directors and designated physicians are ER physicians, there may also be times when they are too busy seeing patients in the ER to speak with the paramedic on the phone.

## OFFLINE MEDICAL DIRECTION

In most, if not all EMS systems in Canada, paramedics are able to perform a limited number of controlled acts and treat the majority of common emergencies under **standing orders**. These medical directives are written in advance and describe medical conditions and prescribe drugs or medical procedures that the paramedic may perform without direct consultation with a physician. This allows for immediate treatment of common emergencies in the field without the delay of using a telephone, radio, or other communication devices.

Offline medical directives generally contain the following information:

▓ description of a medical condition, primary problem, or chief complaint

▓ statement that physician contact is not necessary

▓ the drug or procedure to be administered

▓ the conditions that must be present to carry out the standing order (e.g., minimum patient age, weight, vital sign parameters)

▓ contraindications to the drug or procedure

▓ an algorithm describing the proper sequence of events (e.g., establish an intravenous line prior to administering a particular drug)

# PARAMEDIC LEVELS

One of the most exciting things to happen in recent EMS history was the development by PAC of the Canadian National Occupational Competency Profiles (NOCP) in 2001 (see Appendix C).[10] They were developed on a mandate from Human Resources and Skills Development Canada (HRSDC), formerly HRDC, to dismantle the barriers to paramedic reciprocity across Canada. Led by Project Director Mary Beth Gibbons, this was one of the most ambitious endeavours in Canadian EMS history. Paramedics, paramedic educators, medical directors, ambulance service providers, the Canadian Forces, and other stakeholders spent 3 years developing a consensus on paramedic practitioner levels and a set of competency profiles for each. Many training programs across Canada participate in the voluntary national accreditation process of the Canadian Medical Association (CMA). The CMA's *Requirements for Accreditation* include the expectation that program graduates will possess the competencies outlined in the NOCPs. This not only enhances job mobility for paramedics but has also served to promote national consistency in paramedic training and practice.

Three paramedic practitioner levels—primary care, advanced care, and critical care—were established to meet the needs of all patients and the operational requirements of ambulance services. An additional level, emergency medical responder (EMR) level, was established for volunteers with rural and remote ambulance services who do not have the means to be trained as fully qualified paramedics. This level of advanced first-aid training is also useful for firefighters, who respond to a number of calls alongside paramedics, for industrial workers providing first aid, and for other first responders.

Education for primary, advanced, and critical care forms a continuum. As with other healthcare disciplines, it is important that initial paramedic education set the foundation for further learning. This requires a solid grounding in health sciences and in other essential educational elements.

A Primary Care Paramedic should have a broad and deep enough knowledge base so that the next levels of paramedic education require only a review of such subjects as human anatomy, physiology, and pathophysiology.

## Primary Care Paramedic

**Primary Care Paramedics (PCPs)** make up the vast majority of full-time and part-time paramedics working in EMS systems in Canada. These are career paramedics associated with urban, suburban, rural, remote, air ambulance, and military services. They receive a foundational education solidly based in the health sciences, social sciences, reading, professional writing, numeracy, oral communication skills, thinking skills, and the use of computer technologies. In addition, PCPs are expected to demonstrate excellent decision-making skills, based on sound knowledge and principles. They are also trained to make a differential diagnosis, infer a provisional diagnosis, and implement a management plan, which may include the use of a limited number of controlled medical acts (see Box 1-1), including semi-automated defibrillation and the administration of select medications.

## Advanced Care Paramedic

**Advanced Care Paramedics (ACPs)** have the knowledge and skills to manage more complex medical and traumatic emergencies. Entry into ACP programs generally requires prior certification at the PCP level or equivalency granted by the provincial or territorial regulatory agency. Like PCPs, ACPs are primarily career paramedics. In many parts of Canada, ACPs are paired with PCPs on ambulances to ensure that the maximum number of patients can receive an advanced level of care when needed. In addition to holding PCP competencies, ACPs can carry out an increased number and variety of controlled medical acts. They are trained in advanced procedures, including endotracheal intubation, surgical airway management, needle decompression of the chest in tension pneumothorax (collapsed lung), intravenous drug administration, and various electrical therapies for life-threatening heartbeat irregularities.

## Critical Care Paramedic

Certification as a **Critical Care Paramedic (CCP)**, the highest currently available, requires successfully completing a recognized educational program at the critical-care level. CCPs make up a small number of specialized paramedics in Canada, and most work in the aeromedical industry, providing critical care to patients in flight. A smaller number of CCPs work on land-based critical-care transportation units. In addition to the PCP and ACP knowledge base and **scope of practice**, CCPs work at a level similar to that required in a hospital intensive care unit. CCPs are trained to interpret laboratory and radiological data and to perform controlled acts over and above the ACP level. CCPs work with highly sophisticated medical equipment, including complex **mechanical ventilators** and **hemodynamic monitoring devices**. CCPs typically implement invasive and pharmacological treatment measures.

The competencies at each practitioner level are cumulative: each level includes and exceeds the competencies of the previous level. Most educational institutions require that paramedics gain experience in the field before returning to school to pursue the next level of certification.

## BECOMING A PROFESSIONAL PARAMEDIC

In Canada, standards for paramedic programs are set at the provincial or territorial level. Before 2001, the disparity across the country was significant. In the few years since the introduction of the NOCP, Canadian paramedic educators have come a long way toward achieving nationwide standards. Although some disparities in educational programs remain, the gaps are narrowing, and educators are sharing views, expertise, and innovative ideas more than ever before.

## Certification

Typically, after completing the required education, a paramedic undergoes testing to achieve certification. Certification is a process by which a provincial or territorial ministry of health or branch agency recognizes the competence of the graduate paramedic. Certification may also be granted by a

---

**BOX 1–1    Examples of Controlled Medical Acts as Defined by the Ontario Health Professions Regulatory Advisory Council (HPRAC)**

1. Communicating to the individual or his or her personal representative a diagnosis identifying a disease or disorder as the cause of symptoms of the individual in circumstances in which it is reasonably foreseeable that the individual or his or her personal representative will rely on the diagnosis.
2. Performing a procedure on tissues below the dermis, below the surface of a mucous membrane, in or below the surface of the cornea, or in or below the surface of the teeth, including the scaling of teeth.
3. Moving the joints of the spine beyond the individual's usual physiological range of motion using a fast, low amplitude thrust.
4. Setting or casting a fracture of a bone or a dislocation of a joint.
5. Administering a substance by injection or inhalation.
6. Putting an instrument, hand or finger
   • beyond the external ear canal,
   • beyond the point in the nasal passages where they normally narrow,
   • beyond the larynx,
   • beyond the opening of the urethra,
   • beyond the labia majora,
   • beyond the anal verge, or
   • into an artificial opening into the body.
7. Applying or ordering the application of a form of energy prescribed by the *Regulated Health Professionals Act*.
8. Prescribing, dispensing, selling or compounding a drug as defined in subsection 117 (1) of the *Drug and Pharmacies Regulation Act*, or supervising the part of a pharmacy where such drugs are kept.
9. Prescribing or dispensing for vision or eye problems, subnormal vision devices, contact lenses or eye glasses other than simple magnifiers.
10. Prescribing a hearing aid for a hearing impaired person.
11. Fitting or dispensing a dental prosthesis, orthodontic or periodontal appliance or a device used inside the mouth to protect teeth from abnormal functioning.
12. Managing labour or conducting the delivery of a baby.
13. Allergy challenge testing of a kind in which a positive result of the test is a significant allergic response.

designated base hospital. The base hospital's medical director authorizes the paramedic to perform controlled acts.

## Registration

Registration is the process by which a province or territory grants a paramedic who meets the requirements for safe, optimal patient care the designation to practise. Requirements may include, in addition to certification as a paramedic, a clean driving record, no criminal record and Canadian citizenship.

## Licensure

Licensure is an official form of permission granted to a professional under a *Regulated Health Professions Act (RHPA)*. At this time, only Alberta has a regulated professional body of paramedics. That is not to say that other Canadian paramedics are not regulated, in the less official sense of the term. In fact, one might argue that paramedics in some provinces or territories are the most regulated "unregulated" healthcare professionals on the planet. Standards of care are overseen by the provincial or territorial ministry of health, a ministry-designated base hospital and medical director, and the ambulance service provider for whom they work.

## Reciprocity

Canada's Agreement on Internal Trade (AIT) requires provinces and territories to facilitate the transfer of professionals from one part of Canada to another. **Reciprocity** is the process by which a province or territory grants permission for professionals from another province or territory to practise. Notwithstanding the AIT, when a paramedic moves from one place to another, the province or territory will review his or her credentials and may elect to screen the candidate through written and practical assessments. The purpose of these assessments is not to block the candidate from entering but to do a gap analysis to see if any additional skills training or education is needed to allow for a smooth transition.

## Continuing Medical Education

The field of health care, whether in paramedicine, nursing, respiratory therapy, or any other discipline, is extraordinarily dynamic. Thousands of new drugs and procedures are introduced annually. Medical research continually questions the efficacy of what practitioners do and asks, "How can we do it better?" This means that the paramedic's scope of practice will continually evolve and improve. To keep pace and maintain competence and proficiency, paramedics must engage in continuing medical education (CME). CME may take many forms, including attending seminars, skills review workshops, certificate courses, and medical rounds where real patient care cases are discussed.

Paramedics must be responsible and accountable for their own CME and must commit to a path of lifelong learning.

## Professionalism

Paramedics are not only held accountable to a high level of care; they are also given a privileged trust to meet people's needs at an extremely vulnerable point in their lives. They are welcomed into the privacy of people's homes and allowed to get close in a way few others are. Paramedics are ambassadors of the profession and of the service that employs them. For these reasons, their behaviour must be beyond reproach.

Paramedics must always be in a state of readiness. This means, for example, that on arriving at work, they must take care of business first before socializing or relaxing with colleagues. Vehicle checks, medical equipment checks, cleaning, and stocking are just some examples of duties that take priority.

Paramedics must do more than provide good patient care. They must be kind and respectful to patients, their families, colleagues, and other emergency services personnel. They must be reliable, responsible, and accountable for all of their duties, including keeping their medical knowledge current.

Paramedics must be equally good at giving and taking direction. This requires a balance of confidence, leadership, and humility. These are the traits that make the paramedic an asset to the service and a pillar of the community.

## Desirable Attributes of the Professional Paramedic

In a recent study conducted in the United Kingdom, a panel of EMS experts developed a consensus on desirable qualities in ambulance personnel.[11] In total, 36 attributes were ranked in order of desirability; interestingly, knowledge and skills did not rank in the top five. In fact, clinical skills ranked fourteenth. The results of the study are a testament to the importance of attitude over aptitude. While aptitude is essential, attitude and strength of character are what make an employee an indispensable asset to the paramedic service. The top-five desirable attributes, as determined by Kilner, are

- honesty;
- a patient-centred approach;
- caring, empathy, and valuing life;
- professionalism; and
- a nonjudgmental and nondiscriminatory attitude.[11]

### HONESTY

Honesty comes in many forms. It comes in the form of being truthful to family, friends, colleagues, employers, and the patients we encounter on a day-to-day basis. The public bestows upon us a sacred trust. They allow us to come into their homes, into their workplace, and into their lives; they share with us their most intimate personal information. In return, they expect us to be law-abiding, trustworthy, and respectful of their privacy and their dignity. They expect us to be candid with them when they ask questions about their condition, and honest enough to admit to what we do not know.

Another important element of honesty is being accountable for our actions and our shortcomings. It means not blaming others or circumstances for errors we may make in the field, or for deficiencies in our knowledge base or decision-making abilities. Honesty means going to our supervisor, manager, or medical director when we believe we have made an error in patient care, rather than waiting for someone else to discover the error.

## PATIENT–CENTRED APPROACH

In the beginning of a paramedic's career, it is natural to be nervous about responding to calls. What will you see? Will you be overwhelmed by the sight of grotesque injuries? Being patient-centred means keeping in perspective that your fears pale by comparison to the patient's.

If you attended to calls and you found yourself wondering what others thought of your performance or whether they would later sing your praises, you would be described as self-centred. If you attended to calls and you found yourself wondering what others thought of your performance and worried that they were judging you or might think negatively of your performance, you would also be self-centred. Whether a self-centred approach is rooted in arrogance or insecurity, the patient becomes secondary.

Being patient-centred means focusing on the patient, and determining the patient's needs from his or her perspective, not yours. It means trying to comprehend the patient's fear, anxiety, pain, and perception of events without filtering and without making assumptions. It also means providing patients with the care *they* need. You may sometimes be tempted to provide some aspect of care, such as starting an intravenous, just because you can or because the patient's condition vaguely meets a set of criteria. It is important to keep in perspective at all times that out-of-hospital care is not about you; it is about the patient.

## CARING, EMPATHY, AND VALUING LIFE

No one can deny that patient care skills are an essential and important prerequisite to good paramedic practice, but whether you provide average care or exceptional care, what the patient and family will remember when you leave is whether you communicated with them in a kind and caring manner.[12] In fact, the most common complaints made against paramedics concern attitude and efforts made to meet the patient's needs.[12]

Caring can be defined in many ways, but in the context of health care, it means helping other individuals regain and maintain control and balance in their time of crisis. Sometimes, all that is needed is to demonstrate empathy through listening and acknowledging their anxieties.

Caring also means providing rapid and competent medical care without judgment and without reservation.

Valuing life demands that paramedics reflect on their own values and beliefs to ensure that they do not interfere with the ability to render care without bias or prejudice of any kind. Paramedics must be able to respect and value *all life* even if at times another person's lifestyle, beliefs, values, or behaviour may seem objectionable or even repulsive.

## PROFESSIONALISM

Professionalism in the formal sense of the word refers to "owning" a specialized body of knowledge, belonging to a regulatory body or professional group, strictly adhering to standards and codes of conduct, and being accountable to the public. In a less formal sense of the word, professionalism means many things to different people. However, common themes include appearance and personal hygiene, integrity, respect for all life, accountability, diplomacy, commitment to one's profession, commitment to maintaining personal competence, and willingness to share knowledge with new colleagues entering the field.

## NONJUDGMENTAL AND NONDISCRIMINATORY ATTITUDE

Being a paramedic requires the ability to provide patient care without judgment or discrimination based on race, national or ethnic origin, colour, religion, gender, sexual orientation, age, or mental/physical disability.[13] It requires **cultural competence**, tolerance, and the discipline to focus on the medical needs of the patient.

Being nonjudgmental also means being mature enough to accept that when you encounter a patient, family member, or bystander who is hostile toward you, it has nothing to do with you personally. This is where caring and empathy are most powerful in getting through the layers of hostility to the root cause of the behaviour. Poise, professionalism, and a nonjudgmental approach almost always yield positive results. Take an everyday example of an incident of "road rage," which begins when one driver inadvertently cuts off another. The initial reaction of the first driver might be remorse. But when the other driver begins shouting obscenities, the first returns the shouting, and the two begin a senseless and reckless battle of wits that ultimately endangers their lives and the lives of other drivers. Had the first driver remained true to the initial feeling of remorse and given the other driver an apologetic look or a nonconfrontational gesture, the incident would likely have been defused immediately.

In your career, you will encounter many people who will be verbally and sometimes physically abusive with no provocation whatsoever. Your perception will determine your reaction, and your reaction will determine the outcome. Maturity, compassion, professional poise, and a patient-centred approach will defuse the vast majority of potentially hostile situations.

# PARAMEDIC SUBSPECIALTIES

Although an ambulance of some kind is the conventional setting for paramedics to perform their duties, there is a rapidly emerging interest in how paramedics can best meet the needs of *all* patients in a given area, rather than simply those that can be conventionally accessed. Special situations call for specialized teams. In a hostage-taking situation, for example, the traditional approach would have been for paramedics to remain at a safe distance from the scene and wait for the wounded to be brought to them by the police. With specialty training, tactical paramedics can enter hostile situations under police cover and provide immediate care to the wounded.

Special paramedic response capabilities vary from community to community. To justify the expenditure of time, money, and resources, a paramedic special unit must meet an actual or perceived need. Units should be designed to deal only with events that have a reasonable probability of occurring. Thus, a special unit that makes sense for one community might not be appropriate for another.

The number and variety of paramedic special operations continue to grow. Some of these teams are unique to EMS, while others require interagency partnerships with allied emergency and protective services. The creation of such teams is limited only by the balance that must be struck between having a creative vision and maintaining fiscal responsibility to the taxpayer. This section, then, is not an exhaustive listing but merely a sampling of some of the more common special operations in Canada.

## Tactical Paramedic Support Teams

Tactical emergency medical support is "the comprehensive out-of-hospital medical support of law enforcement's tactical teams during training and special operations."[14] Hundreds of special weapons and tactics (SWAT) teams throughout the world now possess this lifesaving resource, but it is still relatively new to Canada. The first such Canadian team originated in Toronto in 1996.

With appropriate training and equipment, specially trained tactical paramedics can move much closer to support police operations at situations involving shootings, hostage taking, barricaded subjects, or high-risk warrant service. Without tactical paramedics, innocent victims would have to wait until the scene was completely secured or until they could be brought outside a designated perimeter.

Ballistics and weapons familiarization is typically part of this training, although unlike many U.S. teams, Canadian tactical paramedics are generally not armed. Instead, they rely for their personal safety on the police officers with whom they train closely (see Figure 1–2).

Tactical paramedics must be physically fit, exceptionally good team players, and able to follow commands without question. This hierarchy of command is significantly different from the everyday independence paramedics are accustomed to, and it takes great discipline to stay focused on the safety of the team when injured civilians may be nearby and calling for help. Training focuses on adapting prehospital care for delivery in a high-risk environment. The differences from conventional operations must be learned and practised.

Other training focuses on more specific tactical operations and concepts and on safely integrating the paramedic into the team. Topics of training typically include understanding tactical team operations, cover, and concealment; recognizing explosives and booby traps; operating near clandestine drug operations; the use of pyrotechnics, chemical munitions (such as pepper spray and tear gas), and respirators (gas masks); less-than-lethal-use-of-force options (such as the TASER®); crime scene preservation; and modified means of safely accessing, extricating, and managing injured people during a high-risk incident. In some areas of the country, there may be further subspecialization, such as providing paramedic support at political protests, crowd situations, riots, and other civil disturbances.

Incidents such as the shootings at the Columbine High School in the United States all too clearly illustrate the potential need for tactically trained paramedics. However, extremely violent events are not unique to the United States; nor are they limited exclusively to large municipal centres. Following a rage shooting at a bus garage in Ottawa, a Coroner's jury made four recommendations of specific relevance to EMS,[15] which are often quoted to justify the development of tactical EMS capability in Canadian communities.

## Chemical, Biological, Radiological, Nuclear (CBRN) Teams

In the aftermath of the terrorist attacks of September 11, 2001, in the United States, the federal government of Canada, as well as some municipalities acting independently, began to more thoroughly assess the need for a capability to intervene in a terrorist CBRN event. Highly specialized CBRN teams exist in Canada's larger population centres and key border areas. Ideally they are multidisciplinary units comprising forensic specialists, bomb technicians, hazardous materials (HazMat) technicians, and paramedics. Their aim is the capacity to "intervene to mitigate and neutralize an incident and take direct action to save lives."[16] They are trained both locally and nationally.

Paramedics specifically trained to support a CBRN team learn about the characteristics and identification of weapons of mass destruction, the use of personal protective equipment (PPE) and detection instruments, and how to work with a multidisciplinary team in high-risk situations.

## Hazardous Materials Paramedics

Calgary was the first Canadian centre to train paramedics specially to deal with general hazardous materials incidents, such as those seen in chemical factories or in transportation

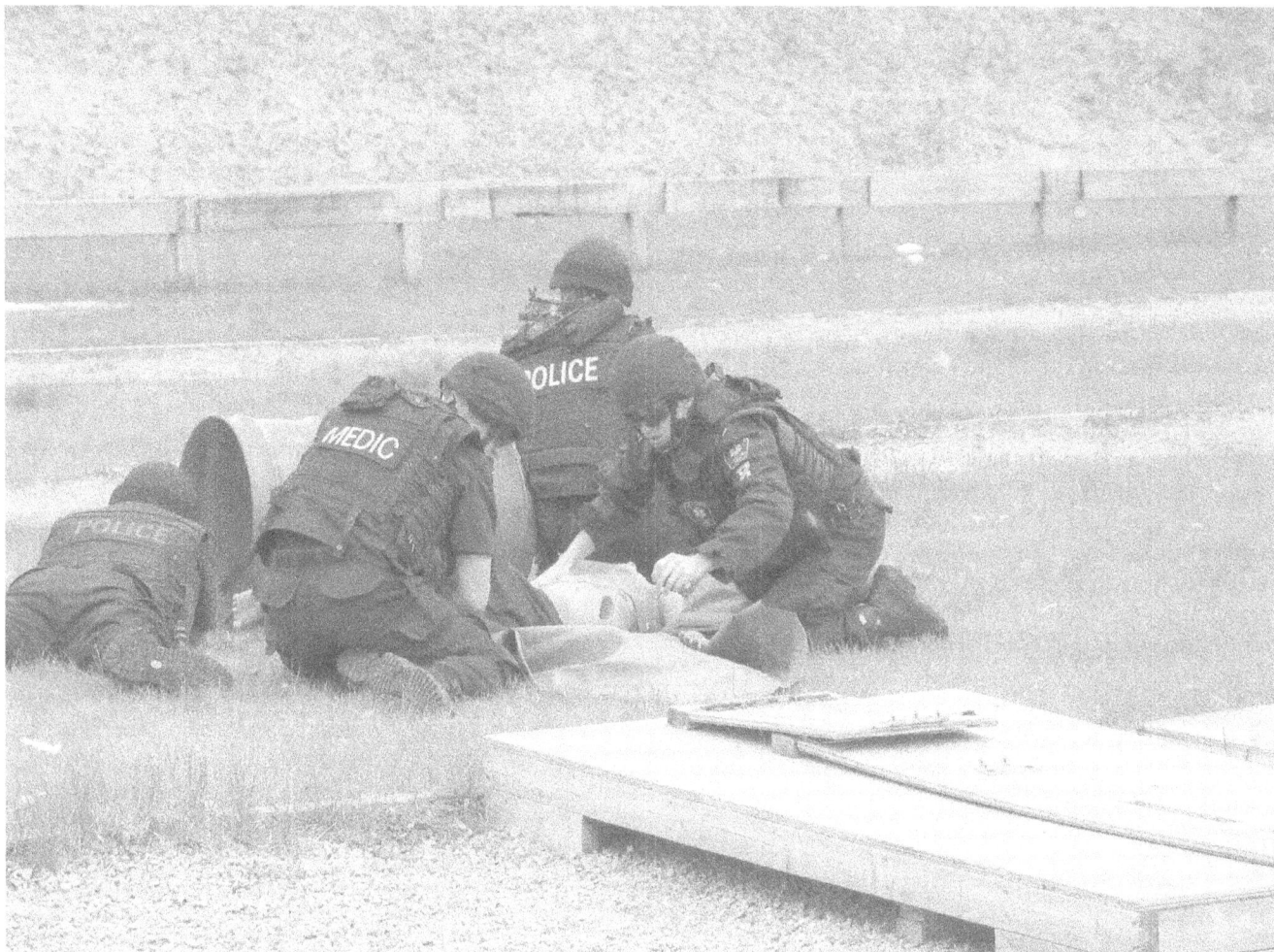

FIGURE 1–2  A mock tactical exercise in Hastings-Quinte.

of dangerous goods. The first 20 HazMat paramedics graduated in April of 2002.[17] Following their success, a second such team was developed with the Hastings-Quinte EMS in Hasting County, Ontario (see Figure 1–2).

Such teams brief paramedic supervisors and staff on the appropriate level of PPE and safety precautions required, anticipated patient symptoms, and the treatment or antidotes for patients exposed. They provide appropriate general or specific care for victims of HazMat incidents and work alongside fire department and HazMat experts to provide preventive and safety-related medical assistance during HazMat operations.

Two main fields typically characterize training: HazMat operations and medical support. HazMat operations training is more technical and includes topics such as putting on and taking off chemical protective suits, respirators, and self-contained breathing apparatus; understanding HazMat product and container research; determining methods of decontamination; assessing medical threats; and conducting HazMat scene survey and safety operations. Training for specific medical support is geared to a more thorough understanding of toxicology, use of a limited range of antidotes, medical monitoring of responders, and general safety-related scene management considerations.

## Paramedic Bike Teams

Many EMS agencies use bicycles for first response. Bicycle teams may be deployed in areas where access may be restricted for regular ambulances, such as bike trails, congested outdoor markets, festivals, air shows, airport terminals, parades, outdoor concerts, or other special events. The flight terminals at the Vancouver and Calgary international airports, for example, are staffed with full-time bike paramedics. In some areas, these teams are deployed only when needed, while in others they operate daily in season, for example, in crowded parks and along beaches.

These teams may offer a cost-effective way to get first-response paramedics to the side of a sick or injured person, often more quickly than would be possible for a land ambulance or for paramedics on foot.

The bicycles used, often mountain bikes or hybrids, are usually fitted with saddle-bags carrying a wide variety of basic life support (BLS) and advanced life support (ALS) equipment, up to and including a small supply of oxygen and a compact defibrillator unit. Variations on the first-responder bike paramedic team concept include the use of motorcycles, ATVs, modified golf carts, snow machines, and equestrian units.

## Paramedic Marine Units

Paramedics are establishing an increasing presence in areas known for waterfront sports and recreation. They often work with police- or fire-based marine units. Adding paramedics to such teams offers the ability to rapidly provide a high level of prehospital medical care at a patient's side. Potential patients served by marine paramedics include not only those who have nearly drowned but also lakeside cottagers and recreational boaters experiencing medical emergencies and police divers taken ill or injured during training or an actual operation. As with many EMS special operations units, marine units also project a positive public image and improve public perception of paramedic operations.

Marine paramedics generally undergo extensive aquatics and water rescue training. Subspecialties may include swift-water or river rescue and ice rescue during the winter months.

## Heavy Urban Search and Rescue

Heavy urban search and rescue, or HUSAR, is defined by Emergency Preparedness Canada as "the location of trapped persons in collapsed structures using dogs and sophisticated search equipment; the use of heavy equipment such as cranes to remove debris; the work to breach, shore, remove and lift structural components; the treatment and removal of victims; and the securing of partially or completely collapsed structures."[18] Such teams are highly multidisciplinary in nature and require considerable interagency cooperation and cross-training. At present, HUSAR teams formally exist or are in development in Vancouver, Calgary, Toronto, Halifax, and the province of Manitoba. Light and medium urban search and rescue capabilities are also established in 41 smaller urban centres across the country.[19]

Training typically includes technical rope rescue, emergency building shoring, confined space operations, HazMat operations, trench and excavation rescue, basic K-9 (dog) first aid, technical search operations, logistics functions and operations, and understanding the **incident management system (IMS)**. Naturally, specialization evolves along professional lines, although all members of HUSAR teams undergo some degree of cross-training so as to become familiar with the full range of team capabilities and limitations. In particular, paramedics might receive special training in triage, managing multiple patients, and recognizing and managing crush injuries.

## Emergency Medical Services in the Canadian Forces

In thinking of EMS special operations, people tend to think of civilian operations. But the military has long accepted the predictable challenge of delivering out-of-hospital medical care in less than ideal circumstances. Not surprisingly, when the NOCP project began, the Canadian Forces eagerly participated.

Entry level military medical technicians (privates and corporals) follow a course of training consistent with PCP training; with time and promotions, selected members undergo training consistent with the advanced and critical-care levels. Some will also be trained as physician's assistants, an occupational classification distinct from a classical paramedic role but with many similarities. (This position is currently making inroads into civilian EMS.)

Military medics are employed in clinics, in operational field units, on board ships, and with air force squadrons. Some work in the most remote and austere locations imaginable, both in peacetime at locations such as the remote Arctic station known as ALERT and in theatres of operation such as peacekeeping and peace-support or war operations. Although military medical technicians are considered noncombatants under the Geneva Conventions, those deployed on operations can and do bear arms to defend both their patients and themselves.[20] Their practice has many similarities to that of civilian tactical EMS and other special operations.

## Flight Paramedics

Canada boasts some of the most sophisticated air ambulance operations in the world. Air ambulance systems include rotary-wing (helicopter) and fixed-wing (airplane) operations. Helicopters are generally used for shorter distances and for landing at the scene of an incident. Airplanes, including small turboprop aircraft, small jets, and larger commercial jets, are used to transport patients over greater distances. Patients transported by aircraft may range in medical priority from the vacationer who is recovering from an injury and returning in stable condition with a medical escort onboard a commercial airline, to the critically injured patient who has been involved in a multi-vehicle collision where the helicopter has landed a few metres from the incident.

Flight paramedics are specially trained to work in the turbulent, noisy, and confined space of a small aircraft. They are also extensively educated in the effects of altitude on both patients and crew. This requires a thorough understanding, for example, of the laws of physics that govern the behaviour of atmospheric gases with ascent and descent from altitude. Because of the noise inside a small aircraft, flight paramedics may not be able to use a stethoscope. This and many other unique aspects of the flight environment require the flight paramedic to be adaptable and able to find alternative means of assessing critical patients.

## In-Hospital Paramedic

With dwindling resources and a shortage of doctors and nurses, paramedics in some communities are being hired to work in the hospital setting. Their knowledge and skills are well suited to serve acutely ill or injured patients visiting the emergency department. Their knowledge of acute resuscitation complements the broader knowledge of the emergency-room nurse, and when physician staffing is less than optimal, paramedics help fill the void.

## Public Information Officer or Public Education Officer

Although not specifically engaged in patient care, the public information officer (PIO) or public education officer (PEO) plays a critical role in allowing paramedics, both conventional and specialist, to perform their duties uninterrupted and with the necessary support from both the media and the public.

"If it bleeds, it leads." This is a common phrase used by reporters that explains why many of the incidents paramedics respond to are of interest to the media. Quite simply, an incident that captures the community's attention and is caught on film will often be on the six o'clock news or the front page of the newspaper. The very nature of a paramedic's work makes it of interest to the media: it is an emergency, it is happening in the community, and lives often hang in the balance. So if the media are so interested in the world of EMS, why not let them in to tell the story?

Paramedics do great work every day caring for the sick and the injured in their community. But does the community know about the timely, high-quality, professional medical care provided by their ambulance service? If it does not, it should. Paramedics across Canada are providing a level of medical care on the street, in residences, and in the back of ambulances that in the not-too-distant past were provided only in the controlled environment of the ER or an operating room. It is a level of medical care the community members deserve to receive when they call for help; they also need to know the paramedics are there. The local media are always keen to tell the story.

Reporters scan radio transmissions, race to the scene of major incidents, take pictures or video, and want to interview someone at the scene with the facts. They want someone reliable and credible, with first-hand information on the situation—usually someone in a uniform. The paramedics at the scene of an incident are subject matter experts; they have first-hand experience and are, with rare exceptions, the highest medical authority on site.

There is tremendous value in having someone designated to speak to the media on behalf of paramedics and EMS operations. An increasing number of services have a PIO from within their ranks to represent the organization publicly. Some organizations may not have the financial resources to hire a full time PIO; however, designating a few staff as spokespersons when on duty is also very effective.

Representation by a designated PIO ensures that a consistent message is delivered, policies are followed, and patient confidentiality is not compromised. If paramedics, administrators, or other officers speak to the media, liaising with the PIO in advance can also help prepare for the interview and reduce anxiety.

The PIO can establish credibility by providing accurate and timely information. A reputable PIO is often considered a medical expert by the media and will be contacted for interviews regarding incidents to which paramedics respond. Additionally, reporters may want to interview the PIO for general interest stories such as illness and injury prevention. Every ambulance service in every community can embrace opportunities to be heard and to increase its profile in the community. If reporters cannot get the information from paramedics, they will get it from someone else.

Part of establishing a relationship with the local media is fostering two-way communications. Providing the media with a dedicated phone number they can always use to contact EMS is a must; most use cell phones or pagers for this purpose. Establishing a system to send media releases is equally important. Modern technology provides a variety of options such as fax and e-mail. A wireless laptop or personal digital assistant (PDA) allows a media release to be sent directly from the scene of an incident. This may be easier, and it also provides the information to the media sooner, which can be extremely valuable to a reporter working on a deadline.

A positive relationship with the media and the timely provision of accurate information is part of a philosophy of public accountability. EMS is a public service, often directly accountable to the public, either through city council or a public committee. The public has a right to know how tax dollars are being spent and to know that a front-line emergency medical service is able and prepared. Working with the media in a positive way provides a means to relay strategic messages, ensure a high public presence, and instill public confidence in the service.

For example, we have all heard stories of a sick person who drove to the hospital instead of calling 911. Good news stories, coupled with strategic messages that highlight short response times and a high level of care, can encourage people to call EMS when in need of medical attention. This positive public profile is also good politics. Many services have their annual budgets approved by their city council or public committee. At budget time, a positive public image can be beneficial for budget approval. An ambulance ride-along for an elected official to see first-hand the inner workings of paramedics and the EMS system can also create political goodwill.

The media can be used as a powerful communications tool to relay injury prevention messages. Do not forget about the media at mass casualty incidents. The bigger the incident, the more reporters will be there. Again, having a PIO or designated spokesperson can be valuable, as he or she works with the media and allow the incident commanders to focus on their priorities. The media can let the public know about road closures, request that people avoid certain areas, or assure the community that an incident is under control. Always be certain you are providing factual information; the community or even the country may be watching.

False perceptions of the media are often based on sensationalized movie scenes depicting a ravenous pack of reporters with cameras. In reality, reporters are just people with a job to do. All they really want is a chance to ask some questions and take a few pictures. Rarely, an unscrupulous reporter will write a one-sided story and burn a hard-earned bridge of yours. In these rare cases, a positive public perception will minimize the damage.

Reporters have a never-ending quest for information. Once you start providing information to the media, be prepared for them to come back for more. There are numerous courses devoted to the subject of media relations. After attending a course, many people find that with a little experience, they quickly become comfortable with the media. A media relations policy can also provide guidance in representing EMS publicly.

Do's and Don'ts when dealing with the media:

**DO**
- Take a course in media relations.
- Follow local ambulance policy and procedure.
- Be prepared.
- Be honest.
- Be professional.
- Be factual.

**DO NOT**
- Lie.
- Say "no comment"—this *is* a comment and implies something negative.
- Provide information you are not authorized to provide.
- Provide patient names or other personal information.
- Provide any information that may compromise a police investigation, such as commenting inappropriately on a homicide, child abuse, sexual assault, or cause of a motor vehicle collision.

## PROFESSIONAL ASSOCIATIONS AND POLITICS

Although the need to improve prehospital emergency medical care was recognized in the early 1970s, it is really only in the past 10 or 15 years that the role of paramedics has evolved with tremendous speed. Undoubtedly, new technology, advancing medical research, rising public expectations, and growing demands on Canada's healthcare system will continue to challenge the development of this relatively young profession. Historically, the role of paramedics has been driven largely by governments, employers, and other medical professions. Now paramedics are organizing within professional associations to take responsibility for the future of their profession.

## Professional Associations

The term *association* can have different meanings, depending on the environment in which it is used. In some jurisdictions, labour organizations (unions and employee bargaining groups) are called associations. In other professions, the "association" may be the regulatory body (more often referred to as a "college") responsible for setting and enforcing standards of practice. More commonly within Canada, professional associations exist apart from unions and regulatory bodies to address the interests and concerns of the profession and its clients. PAC is the national organization of prehospital practitioners, representing the professional interests of paramedics and promoting quality patient care.

PAC and its provincial and territorial chapters strive to develop and strengthen and develop the profession and represent the interests of their practitioners in a number of ways. As professional associations, they:
- Promote quality patient care.
- Raise political and public awareness about the role of paramedics.
- Promote the development and potential of paramedics within the healthcare system.
- Provide leadership in professional and social advocacy initiatives.
- Encourage professional development.
- Develop affiliations and network with other healthcare agencies and EMS stakeholders.
- Collaborate closely with provincial and territorial regulatory bodies on issues of mutual concern.
- Keep members informed of EMS issues and trends.

Perhaps the most significant role of professional associations is representing paramedics with a strong and united voice. Each association can play a significant role in the development of our professional future by validating change. Associations serve as a forum for members to interact and debate within the profession and a vehicle to represent paramedics collectively to other healthcare stakeholders, to government, and to the public. Building consensus among member practitioners and representing the professional interests of paramedics as a strong group brings credibility to the profession and promotes change.

## Government Relations— The Politics of Paramedic Practice

Many in the paramedic profession have marvelled at how our colleagues in the police and fire services have been able to influence politicians for the benefit of their professions and the people they serve. Many of us have wondered why paramedics have been left out of so many issues so often.

The simple answer is that we have rarely made ourselves known to politicians, at least in an ongoing and organized manner. In essence, we were never at the table.

The proliferation of professional paramedic associations in Canada was the first major step to solidifying our ability, as a profession, to successfully lobby governments and politicians alike. Labour unions have done and continue to do good work in lobbying for issues that are important to paramedics. Unfortunately, paramedics are not represented as one group but are often represented by different unions in different areas or make up only a small percentage of a larger union that also represents many other workers with competing issues and concerns. The professional paramedic associations, united with their provincial bodies, which are in turn united with their national body, have made the paramedic profession and the patients that we treat their sole focus.

Becoming a member of your professional association demonstrates to politicians that our profession is organized and that associations do speak on behalf of the profession. The PAC, for instance, represents more than 14,000 members. This wide representation gives credibility and weight in meeting with politicians.

Anyone involved in government relations, whether at the municipal, provincial, or national level, needs to be organized. The professional association needs to organize a government relations committee comprising interested paramedics from across the region it represents.

Establishing a government relations committee allows paramedics to respond to politicians and to the issues that arise on a day-to-day basis. This group can also focus on planning for a yearly visit to the provincial legislature, Parliament Hill, or city hall. Such visits are often referred to as "lobby days."

It is important to meet with politicians regularly. Politicians come and go, and they all need to be educated about what paramedics do and how we help patients. Establishing a yearly lobby days event where paramedics from across the region get together and meet with politicians is a great way to ensure regular contact.

Politicians are busy people who meet with a lot of groups. Someone representing a large group of professionals is more likely to obtain a meeting. It is also important to involve paramedics from the ridings represented by a particular politician. Politicians will usually go to great lengths to set up a meeting with a constituent.

Politicians have busy schedules and may have very little time to spend with you. You may be allotted only 15–20 minutes with each person. Limit your conversation to two or three primary issues of concern. Give a brief overview but leave a detailed information package on each issue. Each information package should start with a one-page brief summarizing

1. what the issue is;
2. your association's views on it; and
3. what you would like the politician to do (e.g., write a letter of support to the Minister of Finance and provide the association with a copy of that letter).

All documentation should include information on how to contact your association and where to find more informa-

tion on the issues. For example, provide links to your Web site, or supply a reference list.

After you have invested significant time and money in an annual event, you must have a communications strategy that will do three things:

1. Ensure that there is follow-up with each politician. Send letters of thanks for meeting with you. Also send sample letters of support that they can use or modify. Finally, once you get support, make sure you recognize it by sending a thank-you letter.
2. Ensure that there is follow-up with your membership. Paramedics need to know what is being said to their politicians, and you also need to solicit their support. Messages you bring to politicians will more likely get their support if they are subsequently contacted by paramedics in their ridings who follow up and ask them what their intentions are.
3. Ensure that there is follow-up with the media. Politicians respect the media because they know that it is the single most important way to communicate with the public. When they see that an organization involves the media, they are more likely to take it seriously and follow up on the issues. Similarly, when the association voices its concerns to the media over political actions that are detrimental to paramedics and the patients we treat, politicians recognize that we have political strength.

# IMPROVING SYSTEM QUALITY: TOTAL QUALITY MANAGEMENT

Paramedics are professionals and as such are accountable to the public. People expect paramedics to be well educated and skilled and to deliver care that is current and solidly grounded in medical evidence. To ensure that paramedics are up to the high standards rightfully demanded by the public, the EMS system, including ambulance operators, base hospitals, and other key stakeholders, must engage in quality assurance and quality improvement through **total quality management (TQM)** activities.

Capezio and Morehouse describe TQM as "a management process and set of disciplines that are coordinated to ensure that the organization consistently meets and exceeds customer requirements. TQM engages all divisions, departments and levels of the organization. Top management organizes all of its strategy and operations around customer needs and develops a culture with high employee participation. TQM companies are focused on the systematic management of data in all processes and practices to eliminate waste and pursue continuous improvement."[21]

From a paramedic service perspective, this means involving paramedics, managers, and support staff in the process of evaluating and improving patient care and patient satisfaction. From a broader ambulance operator perspective, this means evaluating all ("total" in TQM)

EMS activities. TQM is a philosophy of continuous improvement, not just maintenance of the status quo.

TQM addresses all levels of operation, from the big picture to the finest detail. If the end goal is to reduce morbidity and mortality and improve patient satisfaction, each element of paramedic care must be continuously evaluated for improvement opportunities. A quality improvement activity for front-line care, for example, might look at a small piece of the bigger EMS puzzle by evaluating various spinal immobilization devices. An ambulance operator might involve paramedics and other experts to help determine which new device provides the greatest degree of immobilization and comfort, reduces pressure points on the skin, can be applied most quickly to reduce on-scene time, is easiest to clean and disinfect, and is the most cost-effective. If you were to brainstorm with a group of peers, you would no doubt be able to come up with several more criteria.

## Quality Assurance

Quality assurance (QA) is an element of TQM and is the process by which paramedic services establish and maintain programs to promote continuing competence. This may include auditing patient care reports to ensure compliance with local, provincial, or territorial medical directives; holding annual training in workplace hazardous materials information systems (WHMIS); providing CPR retraining; and regularly reviewing policies and procedures. Maintaining paramedic competence is the mainstay of a QA Program. Many, if not most, paramedic services, have a manager whose primary role is ensure quality is maintained and improvements to the overall system are sought and implemented.

## Continuous Quality Improvement

**Continuous quality improvement (CQI)** is predicated on the principle that there is always room for improvement. It is another key element of TQM and stems from a commitment to constantly striving to improve operations, processes, and activities in order to meet patient care requirements in the most efficient, effective, and fiscally responsible manner. It is also a process of evaluating the performance of an operation against benchmarks or industry standards and applying this information to improve operations.

An example of a CQI project would be to implement a new evidence-based intervention (e.g., using 12-lead electrocardiograph (ECG) in the field) and to measure results to see whether, in fact, it improved patient outcomes. A positive outcome in this example might be a reduction in the time it takes for the patient to receive treatment. The broader question would be whether using 12-lead ECG in the field leads to a decrease in morbidity and mortality.

## TQM Principles

Virtually all aspects of a TQM program in an EMS system will affect what paramedics do on the front line. Consequently, paramedics have a vested interest in playing a key role in those processes. Even when paramedics are not directly involved at either a committee or organizational level, it is important to reflect on the principles of TQM and incorporate them into our thinking.

The principles of TQM are as follows:
1. Quality can and must be managed.
2. Everyone has a customer and is a supplier.
3. Processes, not people, are the problem.
4. Every employee is responsible for quality.
5. Problems must be prevented, not just fixed.
6. Quality must be measured.
7. Quality improvements must be continuous.
8. The quality standard is defect free.
9. Goals are based on requirements, not negotiated.
10. Life-cycle costs, not front-end costs, should be tracked.
11. Management must be involved and must lead.
12. Plan and organize for quality improvement.

# SUMMARY

- Canadian paramedics should take pride in their history and in the knowledge that the profession is now portable between the provinces and territories.
- The military experience has had a powerful influence on modern EMS systems.
- Paramedics act as the eyes, ears, and hands of the physician in the field, performing life-saving procedures.
- Paramedic practice is evolving rapidly in Canada. In pursuit of professional status, one province, Alberta, has established self-regulation for paramedics, and other provinces and territories will likely follow suit.
- Paramedic practice is coming under increasing scientific scrutiny. This is a positive advancement for the profession and means that out-of-hospital research will help ensure that paramedics provide care grounded in evidence-based medicine (EBM).
- In 2001, the Paramedic Association of Canada established National Occupational Competency Profiles (NOCP) for three paramedic levels: Primary Care Paramedic (PCP), Advanced Care Paramedic (ACP), and Critical Care Paramedic (CCP). An additional level, the emergency medical responder (EMR), was established in recognition that rural and remote ambulance services continue to be largely staffed by volunteers. This level is also suitable for firefighters who respond with paramedics to medical calls.
- The NOCPs are used as the benchmark for accreditation of educational programs by the Canadian Medical Association (CMA).

- The key to survival in the out-of-hospital setting for victims of illness or injury is to maximize the use of all responder resources, including bystanders, emergency medical dispatchers, firefighters, and police. This is frequently referred to as the "chain of survival."
- Ambulance services are regulated at the provincial or territorial level and delivered, for the most part, by municipalities.
- Canada relies heavily on nonparamedic volunteers to staff ambulance services in rural and remote communities.
- Paramedics are authorized to perform controlled medical acts such as medication administration under the authority of a medical director, usually an ER physician.
- Paramedics are given a sacred public trust, and their behaviour must always be beyond reproach.
- There is a rapidly emerging interest in developing special paramedic training to address special situations. The result has been the development of special operations units such as flight; tactical; chemical, biological, radiation, nuclear (CBRN); HazMat; bike; marine, and heavy urban search and rescue (HUSAR).
- Paramedicine is a rapidly evolving and exciting healthcare discipline. As a career path, it demands a willingness to change as the practice of paramedicine changes. It demands a commitment to lifelong learning. It requires constant self-reflection, accountability, leadership, and the willingness to be led.

# WEBLINKS

- Advanced Coronary Treatment (ACT) Foundation of Canada: The ACT Foundation is a national nonprofit organization dedicated to saving lives by establishing CPR training programs in schools across Canada. www.actfoundation.ca
- Canadian Medical Association (CMA): This is an excellent source for continuing medical education, and it also contains a list of accredited paramedic programs in Canada. http://www.cma.ca
- EMS Chiefs of Canada: Paramedic directors and chiefs from across Canada share position papers, job postings,

paramedic news, and other important information. http://www.emscc.ca
- Paramedic Association of Canada (PAC): PAC has more than 14,000 members and is the national voice of paramedicine in Canada. www.paramedic.ca
- Canadian EHS Research Consortium (CERC): This body's mission is to promote high-quality, multidisciplinary research by facilitating paramedic-driven research, information sharing, and linkages among EMS organizations throughout Canada. www.cerc.paramedic.ca

# REFERENCES

1. Barkley KT. *The Ambulance Fully Illustrated: The Story of Emergency Transportation of the Sick and Wounded Through the Centuries.* New York, NY: Exposition Press; 1978.

2. Hanna JA. *A Century of Red Blankets: A History of Ambulance Service in Ontario.* Erin, Ont: Boston Mills Press; 1982.

3. City of Edmonton. Edmonton, Alberta's Capital. EMS History. Available at: http://www.edmonton.ca/portal/server.pt. Accessed July 10, 2006.

4. McNeil E. *Airborne Care of the Ill and Injured.* New York, NY: Springer-Verlag; 1983.

5. British Columbia Ambulance Service. *Your BCAS Paramedics and You "Working Together for Life."* Available at: http://www.healthservices.gov.bc.ca/bcas/. Accessed July 18, 2006.

6. Welsh RC, Ornato J, Armstrong PW. Prehospital management of acute ST-elevation myocardial infarction: A time for reappraisal in North America. *Am Heart J.* 2003; 145(1):1–8.

7. Heart and Stroke Foundation of Canada. *Home is Where The Heart Stops, Finding Answers for Life.* Available at: http://ww2.heartandstroke.ca. Accessed July 18, 2006.

8. Valenzuela TD, Roe DJ, Nichol G, Clark LL, Spaite DW, Hardman RG. Outcomes of rapid defibrillation by security officers after cardiac arrest in casinos. *N Engl J Med.* 2000;343(17):1206–1209.

9. Romanow RJ. *Commission of the Future of Health Care in Canada.* Available at: http://www.hc-sc.gc.ca/english/care/romanow/index1.html. Accessed July 18, 2006.

10. Paramedic Association of Canada. *National Occupational Competency Profiles for Paramedic Practitioners: June 2001 Introduction.* Available at: http://www.paramedic.ca/. Accessed July 1, 2006.

11. Kilner T. Desirable attributes of the ambulance technician, paramedic, and clinical supervisor: Findings from a Delphi study. *Emerg Med J* [serial online]. 2004;21: 374–378. Available at: http://emj.bmjjournals.com/. Accessed July 18, 2006.

12. Kuisma M, Määttä T, Hakala T, Sivula T, Nousila-Wiik T. Customer satisfaction measurement in emergency medical services. *Acad Emerg Med.* 2003;10:812–815.

13. Department of Justice Canada. *Canadian Charter of Rights and Freedoms.* Available at: http://laws.justice.gc.ca/en/charter/. Accessed July 18, 2006.

14. *International Tactical EMS Association (ITEMS).* Available at: http://www.tems.org/. Accessed July 18, 2006.

15. Canadian Critical Incident Incorporated. *Excerpts from January 2000 Coroner's Inquest.* Available at: http://www.commandpost.tv/octranspo.asp. Accessed July 18, 2006.

16. Public Safety and Emergency Preparedness Canada. *Canadian Emergency Preparedness College CBRN Training Program.* Available at: http://ww3.psepc-sppcc.gc.ca/ep/college/cepc_broch_e.asp#cbrn. Accessed July 18, 2006.

17. City of Calgary, Emergency Medical Services. *Hazardous Materials Paramedics.* Available at: http://www.calgary.ca/portal/server.pt/gateway/PTARGS_0_2_771_203_0_43/http%3B/content.calgary.ca/CCA/City+Hall/Business+Units/Emergency+Medical+Services/Operations/Hazardous+Materials+Paramedics.htm. Accessed July 18, 2006.

18. Toronto Emergency Medical Services. *Heavy Urban Search and Rescue (HUSAR) Overview.* Available at: http://www.toronto.ca/ems/operations/husar.htm. Accessed July 18, 2006.

19. *Public Safety and Emergency Preparedness Canada: Urban Search and Rescue Program.* Available at: http://www.psepc-sppcc.gc.ca/prg/em/usar/index-en.asp. Accessed July 18, 2006.

20. Department of National Defence. *Canadian Forces Recruiting (Medical Technician—A Career as a Non-Commissioned Member).* Available at: http://www.recruiting.forces.gc.ca/engraph/career/tradeinfo_e.aspx?id=737&bhcp=1. Accessed July 18, 2006.

21. Capezio P, Morehouse D. *Taking the Mystery out of TQM: A Practical Guide to Total Quality Management.* Franklin Lakes, NJ: Career Press, 1995.

# 2 Injury Prevention and Health Promotion

## OBJECTIVES

*Upon completion of this chapter, the paramedic student will be able to:*

1. Identify the paramedic's roles in injury prevention and health promotion.
2. Describe the epidemiology of injury in Canada and around the world.
3. Outline the aspects of paramedic practice that makes it a desirable resource for involvement in community health activities.
4. Describe community leadership activities that are essential to enable paramedics to participate actively in community wellness activities.
5. Evaluate statistical data to determine where paramedics can be most effective in reducing injury and promoting health.
6. Differentiate among primary, secondary, and tertiary prevention activities.
7. Describe strategies to implement a successful injury-prevention program.
8. Describe how to measure the effectiveness of injury-prevention and health-promotion activities.

## KEY TERMS

## INJURY EPIDEMIOLOGY

While the world prepares for the next flu pandemic, a more persistent, predictable, and insidious pandemic is sweeping the planet. The name of this pandemic is "preventable injury." The inoculation is heightened injury awareness. The objective from a human behavioural perspective is to positively alter perception so that people accept that risk is an everyday part of their lives but change the way in which they perceive and react to risk to reduce injury.

Worldwide, injury is the leading cause of death and disability between birth and age 59.[1] Road traffic injuries alone are listed as the ninth leading cause of death and disability worldwide for all ages, and the World Health Organization (WHO) predicts it will rank third by the year 2020, just two below ischemic heart disease (see Table 2–1).[2]

In Canada, injuries are the leading cause of death for people aged 1 to 44.[3] In 1999, there were 13,750 deaths due to unintentional injury in all age groups.[3] Injury is ranked the fifth leading cause of death in *all* ages after cancers, heart disease, cerebrovascular disease, and chronic obstructive pulmonary disease.[4] Males are more likely than females to sustain injuries; in 2001, 15.5% of males and 11.1% of females suffered injuries.[5] The cost to the Canadian economy for unintentional injuries alone is estimated at $8.7 billion annually.[6]

Deaths due to injury are merely the tip of the iceberg. For every death, there are 1,500 visits to the ER for treatment and 45 hospital admissions.[3] Currently, injury is the leading cause of potential years of life lost (PYLL) in Canada before the age of 70.[3] Thousands of Canadians are permanently blinded, disabled by brain injury, or paralyzed by spinal cord injury. The devastation of their injuries makes many of them dependent on others for the things most of us take for granted, such as feeding, dressing, performing basic bodily functions, mobility, and day-to-day activities. The emotional toll on those who are severely disabled and their families is incalculable.

## Injury Concepts

*Mosby's Paramedic Textbook* defines injury as intentional or unintentional damage to the person resulting from acute exposure to various forms of energy or the absence of such essentials as heat and oxygen (p. 43).[7] More specifically, it is the cellular damage that occurs as the result of the transfer of energy or the absence of one or two essential elements needed to sustain cellular life. The five types of energy responsible for injury are thermal, radiation, electrical, chemical, and kinetic (TRECK). The two essential elements that are required to prevent injury are oxygen (the absence of which results in suffocation or drowning) and heat (the absence of which results in hypothermia or frostbite).

## Causes of Injury in Canada

### FALLS

Falls are the most common cause of injury in all age groups (see Table 2–2). However, any experienced paramedic realizes that the number of calls for seniors who have fallen is particularly high. In fact, fall-related injuries are nine times as great among seniors as among those under the age of 65.[8] As many as 25% of seniors who experience a fall will sustain a serious injury, such as a fracture.[8] More than 90% of all hip fractures in people over the age of 65 are due to falls, and a staggering 20% will die within a year of the fracture.[8]

Injuries among seniors are debilitating for those who are injured. Moreover, because injuries rob them of their independence, their families are frequently faced with the difficult task of caring for them. Families that rely on two incomes to maintain a mortgage and to care for their children may find the task impossible. Thus, as many as 40% of all nursing home admissions occur after a senior has sustained an injury in a fall.[8]

In 1995, the Canadian healthcare system spent more than $980 million to cover the direct cost of medical care for falls among seniors.[3] As Canada's population ages, without a comprehensive injury-prevention strategy, those numbers will increase.

Children also commonly sustain injuries from falls in day-to-day play in playgrounds and at home (see Figure 2–1). The cost to Canadians for injuries related to childhood falls is approximately $630 million per year.[9]

### MOTOR VEHICLE COLLISION

Canadians rely very heavily on motor vehicles for transportation across more than 900,000 kilometres of roads. Canadians love their automobiles: there are almost 19 million vehicles for a driving population of approximately 21 million.[9]

Motor vehicle collisions (MVCs) are the second leading cause of hospitalization due to injury in Canada.[3,10,11] Approximately 3,000 people die in MVCs each year.[9] To put that into perspective, about eight people die on Canadian roads and highways on an average day. It is the leading cause of premature death and long-term disability.[9] Disturbingly, 40% of all collisions involve alcohol, despite the efforts of private and government agencies to discourage drinking and driving.[3]

Paramedics themselves are particularly vulnerable to MVCs. Most paramedics spend a significant amount of

---

**TABLE 2–1** Change in Rank Order of DALYs* for the 10 Leading Causes of the Global Burden of Disease

| 1990 | | 2020 | |
|---|---|---|---|
| **Rank** | **Disease or Injury** | **Rank** | **Disease or Injury** |
| 1 | Lower respiratory infections | 1 | Ischemic heart disease |
| 2 | Diarrheal diseases | 2 | Unipolar major depression |
| 3 | Perinatal conditions | 3 | Road traffic injuries |
| 4 | Unipolar major depression | 4 | Cerebrovascular disease |
| 5 | Ischemic heart disease | 5 | Chronic obstructive pulmonary disease |
| 6 | Cerebrovascular disease | 6 | Lower respiratory infections |
| 7 | Tuberculosis | 7 | Tuberculosis |
| 8 | Measles | 8 | War |
| 9 | Road traffic injuries | 9 | Diarrheal diseases |
| 10 | Congenital abnormalities | 10 | HIV |

*DALY: disability-adjusted life year. A health-gap measure that combines information on the number of years lost from premature death with the loss of health from disability; HIV: human immunodeficiency virus.
Source: Peden M, Scurfield R, Sleet D, et al., eds. *World Report on Road Traffic Injury Prevention: Summary*. World Health Organization; 2004, p.16.

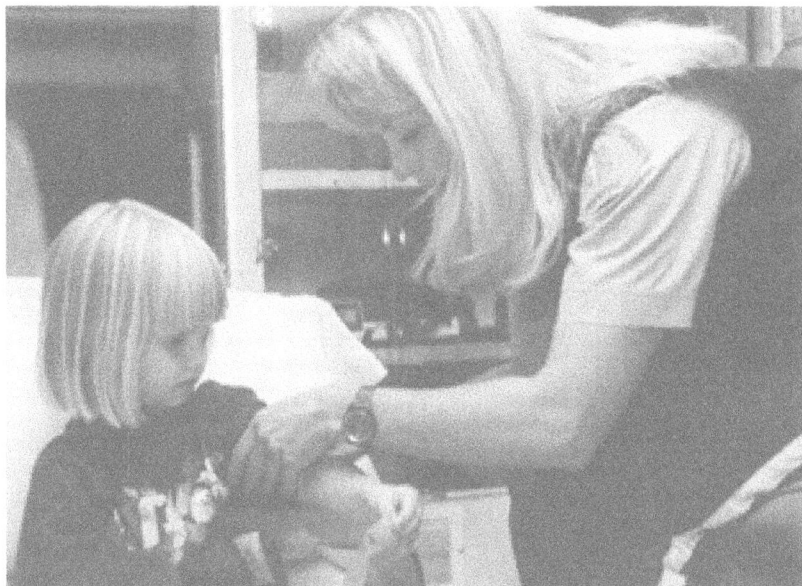

**FIGURE 2–1** A Calgary paramedic looks after a child.

time driving an ambulance or some other vehicle. Not only do they log a tremendous number of hours on the road but they also engage in high-risk driving, exceeding speed limits with the use of lights and sirens. This is not without consequence. In a U.S. study published by *Annals of Emergency Medicine*, line-of-duty deaths (LODD) among paramedics were comparable with those of police officers and firefighters. Paramedics have a rate of 12.7 fatalities per 100,000 workers annually, compared with 14.2 and 16.5 fatalities per 100,000 for police and firefighters, respectively.[12] Seventy-four percent of LODDs in the paramedic field resulted from motor-vehicle-related incidents.[12] In this study, 36% of those who died were driving, 24% were riding in the vehicle, and 27% were caring for patients.[12]

## AGRICULTURAL INJURIES

Many believe that police officers, firefighters, and paramedics have the most risky occupations. In reality, more farmers are killed or injured annually than all emergency services personnel combined. Each year, in Canada, farming injuries result in approximately 120 deaths and 1,200 ER visits.[3] Deaths of farmers and farm workers represent 13% of all occupational fatalities in Canada.[3] Farming is also one of the few occupations in which children are killed in work-related incidents. Children who are raised on farms naturally learn to work on farms. Sometimes, despite the best efforts of parents, children will attempt to demonstrate their maturity and assert their independence by performing farm duties on their own and without instruction. Sometimes simple childhood curiosity will lead them to experiment with unfamiliar equipment. The Canadian Agricultural Injury Surveillance Project (CAISP) estimates that children under the age of 15 account for approximately 10% of all farm-related fatalities.[13]

## CYCLING

Almost all Canadians ride bicycles or have cycled at some time in their life for transportation, fitness, and recreation. Most Canadian children age 6 to 16 ride bicycles.[14] The Canadian Safety Council reports that the majority of bicycle injuries occur as a result of falls or collisions with stationary objects, other cyclists, or pedestrians and that most bicycle-related injuries occur less than five blocks from the person's home.[14] Although fewer than 20% of bicycle incidents involve motor vehicles, those incidents account for 90% of bicycle-related deaths.[14] Over two thirds of bicycle-related deaths result from head injuries.[14] (See Figure 2–2.)

## DROWNING

From 1991 to 2000, there were close to 6,000 water-related deaths in pools, bathtubs, lakes, and other waterways across Canada.[15] Most of these deaths were drownings. Once again, while the number of deaths is disturbing, they do not paint a complete picture. For the same time period, there were 3,289 hospitalizations for near drownings.[15] Many of these survivors are permanently brain damaged and will never lead a normal life.

**TABLE 2–2** Causes of Injury 1999–2000

| | |
|---|---|
| Falls | 38.7% |
| Motor vehicle collisions | 17.7% |
| Struck by object/person/falling object | 9.9% |
| Cycling | 6.4% |
| All other causes of injuries | 27.3% |

*Causes of Injury Admissions in Canadian Children, 1999/2000.* Canadian Institute for Health Information, National Trauma Registry. [8]

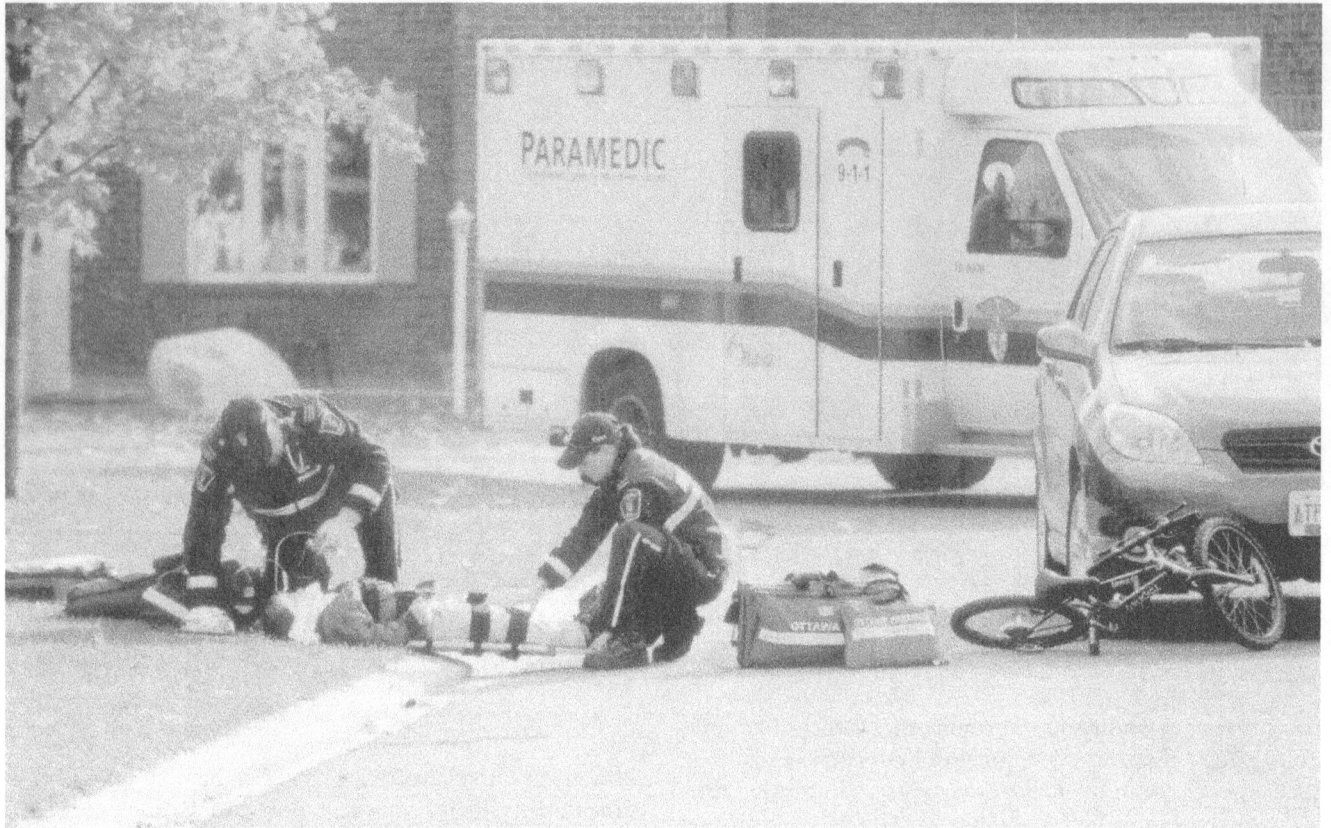

FIGURE 2–2 Ottawa Paramedic Service crew attend to a cyclist struck by a car.

## SNOWMOBILING

Next to water-related injuries, which are accountable for 18% of all serious recreation-related injuries, snowmobiling is close behind at 16%, followed by all-terrain vehicles (13%); downhill skiing (6%); dirt biking, minibikes, and motorcross (5%); horseback riding (5%); and snowboarding (5%).[16]

Snowmobiling is the number-one cause of injuries related to winter recreation in Canada.[17] Injuries sustained in snowmobiling incidents account for 41% of winter-related injuries, followed by snowboarding, skiing, hockey, tobogganing, and ice-skating.[17] Those treated in hospital are most often between the ages of 20 and 39. However, the most seriously injured, who require care at a trauma centre, are more often under 20 years of age.[17]

The majority of snowmobile-related injuries occur on private property (87%), including trails; fewer than 15% take place on roadways.[17] Drivers more often sustain serious injuries than do passengers.[17] Drivers typically are pushed into the dash when the crash occurs; consequently the most common injuries are leg fractures and spinal injuries. Passengers are more likely to be thrown from the snowmobile, which results in fractures and head injuries.[1] According to the most recent data from the Canadian Institute for Health Information, blood alcohol levels are above the legal limit in approximately half of injured snowmobile drivers in whom the blood-alcohol level was recorded.[17] Because blood alcohol levels are not measured consistently, the percentage of impaired drivers may be considerably higher.

## Factors in Injury

There are thousands of mechanisms of injury. The ones described above simply provide a glimpse into some of the more prevalent causes in Canada. For every injury mechanism, a thorough analysis would reveal numerous causative and contributing factors.

## AN OVERVIEW OF INJURY PREVENTION

Prevention begins with an acknowledgment that injury is one of Canada's most serious and most expensive healthcare problems. Injury is not only a tale of human tragedy for those who are injured and their family and friends, it is also a crisis for all Canadians. Taxpayers are all paying the staggering healthcare costs associated with the treatment of injuries on the field, on the surgical table, in the intensive care unit, during rehabilitation, and throughout the life-long assisted care needed by many of those permanently disabled. Everyone is susceptible to injury, and everyone is responsible for prevention.

# Becoming Educated

Whether you plan to participate in or take a leading role in injury prevention, you need to research the injury type you wish to reduce. Your status as a paramedic will give you a certain degree of instant credibility in the public eye; nonetheless, knowing the facts about a particular type of injury issue will be critical to persuading the skeptics in your audience. Some people will also have false beliefs about certain injury causes. It is important to canvass your audience to get a sense of what they know and what they perceive about a particular issue. People who engage in risk-taking behaviour, be it a health matter or an **injury risk**, tend to cling to anecdotes to rationalize their behaviour.

For example, a smoker may be able to name several acquaintances who lived long and healthy lives despite having smoked several packs of cigarettes a day.

A person who drives without wearing a seat belt may try to justify his choice by telling you that he knows of someone who survived a crash only because he was not wearing his seat belt and was ejected to safety. While this may rarely occur, in reality proper use of seat belts reduces the risk of death by 61%.[18] As a paramedic, you can counter with some of your own anecdotes, such as cases in which occupants of a vehicle have been ejected and then struck by other passing vehicles. This is where your knowledge, experience, and credibility may have a persuasive impact.

Some people will tell you that they have a right not to wear a seat belt. They will argue that it is their body and that they can do with it as they please. There are several counterarguments: First, wearing a seat belt is required by law. Second, an occupant who does not wear a seatbelt becomes a projectile and may seriously injure other occupants in the vehicle at the time of the crash. Third, unrestrained occupants are more likely to be seriously injured, and the resulting healthcare costs are a burden shared by all taxpayers.

Another common assertion is that driving at higher speeds on the highway is actually safer. This is a common myth. As reported by the Canadian Safety Council, "as speed increases over 100 km/h, the fatality rate of vehicle occupants goes up exponentially. For example, the chances of being killed in a vehicle travelling at 120 km/h is four times higher than at 100 km/h. When a car crashes near 200 km/h the chances of survival are minimal."[19]

A big part of becoming informed about injury prevention is separating facts from perceptions; changing perceptions can change behaviour. One of the ways to begin to change perception is to change the language used in discussing injury and injury causes. For example, *accident* is the most frequently used word in association with causes of injury. The Canadian Oxford dictionary defines "accident" as "an event that is without apparent cause, or is unexpected…occurrence of things by chance…". By contrast, most injuries are, in fact, predictable and preventable and are therefore not accidents at all.

People cling to the word *accident* because it consoles: "Don't blame yourself, it was an accident." "It couldn't be helped." Most people, for example, would describe a motor vehicle collision as a "car accident." Is it because using any other descriptor might suggest someone is to blame? Perhaps. The word *accident* not only absolves all parties of any blame, it also suggests that there are no identifiable and modifiable factors. In fact, there are many, including driver training, quality of police enforcement, road maintenance or design, highway signage, vehicle design, and tire wear.

Many in the media will use the word *accident* in connection with MVCs. Interestingly, the word *accident* is used far less frequently when describing a plane or train crash. In these instances, there is an immediate assumption that someone or something is to blame. Yet in the everyday occurrences of car crashes people are far more reluctant to assign accountability. Words such as *collision* or *crash* are neutral: they neither lay blame nor absolve anyone of blame; they neither imply causative factors nor dismiss them. Neutral descriptors such as *collision, crash,* or *incident* leave open the opportunity for self-reflection and for identifying a cause or causes so that an injury-prevention strategy can be developed and lives can be saved.

## PUBLIC PERCEPTION OF DISEASE VERSUS INJURY

In one of his many compelling speeches, Dr. Robert Conn, one of the world's leading experts in injury prevention, described the difference in public perception of disease and injury. He suggested that if a school-aged child were to die from meningitis, it would be the top story of almost every television newscast that night, and the next day it would be on the front page of leading newspapers. There would be an outcry from the community and an urgent push for inoculations for all conceivable forms of meningitis. Yet meningitis rarely takes a life. In contrast, there are approximately 38 preventable injury-related deaths each day in Canada. And where is the outcry? The reason for this relative lack of concern, Dr. Conn argued, is that people see diseases such as meningitis as preventable or treatable. On the other hand, people see "accidents" as acts of fate and out of their control.

# Haddon's Matrix

Where do we start when it comes to injury prevention? How do we take an organized approach to ensure that what we do will have a positive and measurable outcome? William Haddon Jr. took a public-health model designed for infectious diseases, adapted it to traffic safety, and called it Haddon's Matrix.[20] The matrix is based on the principle that there is an epidemiology or pattern to injuries—thus, injuries are predictable. Haddon's Matrix has since been adapted and applied by leading injury-prevention organizations for all major injuries.

Since the original development of Haddon's Matrix, there have been several variations designed to more clearly elucidate the complexities of injury causation. One of the

premises of injury prevention is that there are three possible phases in which we may be able to intervene:
■ the pre-event phase;
■ the event phase; and
■ the postevent phase.

Targeting the pre-event phase is described as **primary injury prevention**. The objective is to prevent the event from occurring in the first place. Activities in this area may include training drivers, scuba divers, and sky divers; teaching parents to dress their children in reflective clothing before they go out for Halloween; or teaching teenagers to check the depth of a lake before making a headfirst plunge. Another example is spotting a gymnast to make sure she lands on her feet and not her head. A parent who holds a child's bicycle as he learns to ride for the first time or instructs him to look both ways before crossing the road is engaged in primary injury prevention.

Injury prevention at the event phase (the point at which injury occurs) is known as **secondary injury prevention**. The extent of injury is determined by four factors (see Box 2–1): the type of energy transferred (TRECK); the amount of energy (e.g., speed at the time of impact for kinetic energy, or temperature to which one is exposed for thermal energy); the length of exposure to the energy (e.g., radiation, heat, chemical); and, finally, the protective gear or protective engineering built into the design of inanimate objects to mitigate injury (e.g., PPE, seat belts, air bags)

There are many injury-prevention activities aimed at the event phase. For example, cyclists can wear a helmet to reduce the risk of head injury (see Figure 2–3). Up to 85% of serious head injuries could be prevented by wearing a helmet.[14] Indeed, in 2001 all children under the age of 15 who were killed in cycling incidents were not wearing a helmet.[14] Therefore, an example of a secondary injury-prevention strategy might include passing helmet laws, applying the laws to all age groups, and improving enforcement of those laws. (Currently, some provinces have such laws and others do not; moreover, some provinces' laws apply only to children.)

In planning injury-prevention activities, it is important to understand individuals' motivation. One might ask: Why *don't* all people wear helmets when they cycle? Is it because
■ people are not aware that head injury is the leading cause of death in cyclists?
■ people are not aware of how well a helmet protects the cyclist from sustaining a head injury?

| Box 2–1 | Determinants of the Type and Severity of Injury |

• Type of energy (or absence of essential elements such as oxygen or heat)
• Amount of energy
• Length of exposure to the energy
• Mitigating protection (e.g., fire-retardant material, PPE)

■ the helmets do not fit properly or are uncomfortable or hot?
■ people fear being ridiculed by others when wearing a helmet?
■ parents do not set a good example?
■ since the law applies only to children in some provinces and territories, people perceive cycling without a helmet as a sign of maturity and advanced cycling skill?

The postevent phase is the period after the injury occurs. Injury prevention in the postevent phase is described as **tertiary injury prevention**. There are many opportunities in the immediate, short-term, and long-term period to reduce the ongoing injury and to help improve and accelerate the recovery process. Out-of-hospital care provided by paramedics has the greatest impact in the first few minutes and hours following the injury. For example, immediately following a burn injury, the objective is to cool the burn; as long as the burned area is still hot, the tissue damage will continue and the burn will become deeper and more serious. If someone breaks a leg bone, the objective would be to immobilize the fracture as soon as possible so that the ends of the broken bone do not further damage the surrounding tissues. If someone is knocked unconscious and their flaccid tongue obstructs their airway, rapid intervention will make the difference between life and death.

In the short term, ER interventions followed by surgery can also make the difference between life and death or between a normal life and permanent disability. The long-term rehabilitation process plays an equally important role in accelerating recovery, reducing or preventing disability, and helping the person reintegrate into society.

Tertiary injury-prevention activities might include improving paramedic education and training, adding or improving a medical procedure, or implementing a CQI program for paramedics aimed at shortening the time from injury to surgery.

Given a particular type of injury and mechanism, organizations may focus their energies in one area of prevention or in all three. The ultimate goal of injury prevention would be to completely prevent injuries from occurring in the pre-event phase, thus making the event and postevent phases irrelevant. However, this is not always realistic or practical. For example, preventing all injuries from MVCs would require eliminating all cars, trucks, and other motor vehicles. More achievable primary prevention activities might include better driver training, reducing the incidence of impaired driving, or improving the lighting on roadways.

In addition to the phases of injury, each potential injury also has a *host*, or person at risk of injury; an *agent*, or energy responsible for the injury to the host (thermal, radiation, electrical, chemical, kinetic, or absence of oxygen or heat) through a vehicle (inanimate object) or vector (person or other animal); and an *environment* (e.g., playground, ski hill, roadway, building). The host, agent, and environment are integrated as columns into the Haddon Matrix (see

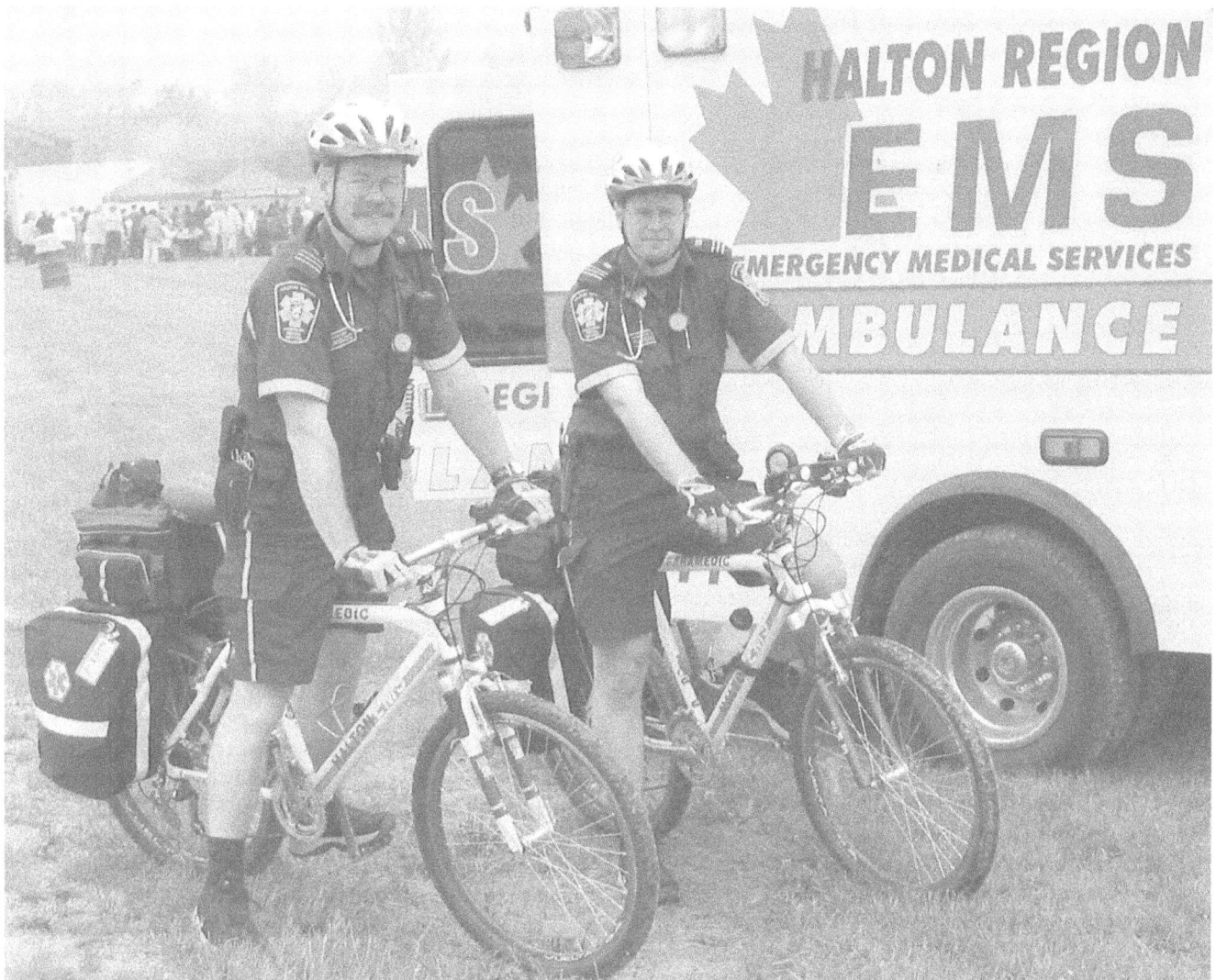

**FIGURE 2–3** Halton EMS bike paramedics wear their protective gear, setting an example for children and adults at a large outdoor event.

Table 3-2 on page 45 of *Mosby's Paramedic Textbook*, 3rd edition). Haddon's matrix demonstrates how injury-prevention activities target the host, agent, or environment in the pre-event, event, and postevent phases.

Let us look at another example of an injury pattern that can be placed into Haddon's Matrix for analysis and evaluation (see Table 2–3). The Canadian Hospitals Injury Reporting and Prevention Program (CHIRPP) revealed that 98% of school injuries treated in hospital for children between the ages of 5 and 9 occur outdoors, and 41% of those injuries occur while children are playing on the monkey bars.[21] In the same study, almost half of the children injured sustained at least one fracture, and 86% of fractures were to the upper extremities.[21] Based on the above information, what additional information would you like to obtain?

One might ask:

▓ Were the upper extremity fractures from contact between the arms and the bars?

▓ Were the upper extremity fractures from contact with the ground after falling from an upside-down position?

Can you think of any other important questions?

## The Three Es of Injury Prevention

Numerous experts and stakeholders play a critical role in injury prevention. Because of the complexity of injury prevention, a multidisciplinary approach will achieve the greatest success, provided it is well organized and includes measurable outcomes in each area. That is, organizers should be able to determine whether the activities actually reduce injury. Injury prevention has traditionally targeted three broad areas, known as the three Es of injury prevention: *education*, *enforcement*, and *engineering*. As the first to see the tragedy of injury, paramedics possess the experience, expertise, and passion to advocate for prevention-oriented activities in all three areas.

**TABLE 2–3** Haddon's Matrix for Playground Injuries

**FACTOR**

| PHASE | HOST | AGENT | ENVIRONMENT |
|---|---|---|---|
| Pre-event | Age, height, familiarity with playground equipment, disability | Defective equipment, height of bar from ground, quality of surface (hard, soft) | Number of children sharing playground equipment, slippery wet surfaces, warning signs |
| Event | Training, protective equipment | ? | ? |
| Postevent | ? | ? | ? |

Try a brainstorming exercise to fill in the blank areas.

## EDUCATION

Education is the area in which paramedics arguably have the greatest opportunity to effect change and reduce injuries. Your status as a paramedic gives you instant credibility in the eyes of the public. Your experience on the front lines will enable you to see risks from a unique perspective.

Education may include:

- Self-education to become aware of the issues, the statistics, and the impact of injury on the injured, the healthcare system, the community, and the broader society.
- Self-education to become aware of who is involved in injury-prevention activity in the community, province, or territory or at a national or international level and of where paramedics can play a role.
- Education of the public to change behaviour and reduce injury.
- Education of other stakeholders in the areas of enforcement and engineering to help them better understand injury from a paramedic and broader healthcare perspective.
- Education of the media to engage them in championing the injury-prevention cause.
- Education of the educators in schools, colleges, and universities to help shape risk perception at all age levels.

Paramedics and other healthcare professionals often think, *If only other people could see what we see, know what we know, and understand the true gravity of injury, they would take fewer risks, and the number of injuries would decline.* From this belief stems a second belief: that if we share our tragic firsthand stories and show our audiences graphic pictures and videos of grotesque carnage, they will be repulsed and frightened into changing their risk-taking ways.

While the experience and the passion that a paramedic brings to the injury-prevention forum are tremendous assets, scare tactics virtually never work.[22] If anything, frightening people drives them further into denial and causes them to cling more tightly to anecdotal references of unbelted car-crash survivors and workers who narrowly escaped head injury because there was no helmet to block their field of vision.

Injury prevention also requires an acknowledgment that risks are a part of everyday life. Whether people take risks for practical purposes, such as transportation to and from work, or for the thrill of sports and leisure activities, it is not possible to eliminate all risks. Nor should we attempt to do so. In the words of Dr. Robert Conn, "risks are what make us feel alive." The objective in injury prevention is to help people become more aware of risks so that they can make informed choices, or take "smart risks." SMARTRISK is, in fact, the name one of the leading injury-prevention organizations in Canada, which is recognized worldwide for its innovative approach to injury prevention. Taking smart risks is a positive approach to injury prevention. Children especially are saturated with the "don'ts" of injury-prevention messages: "Don't cross the street without looking"; "don't go swimming without a buddy"; "don't ride without a helmet." Such messages emphasize deterrents rather than positive incentives. They make wearing protective equipment or following the rules seem tedious. Safety messages aimed at controlling behaviour rather than changing perception are short lived.[22]

The smart-risk approach puts a positive spin on an old message. Whereas taking risks involves acting before thinking, taking smart risks involves first considering the options. For example, "If you ride your bike without a helmet, you're taking a risk without thinking about your options. You're limiting yourself. If you fall, you have a good chance of injuring yourself. But if you choose to take a smart risk and ride with a helmet, you reduce your odds. You have a much greater chance of getting back up on your bike, making it home, and taking another ride the next day."

Taking smart risks allows people to relax and enjoy everyday activities. The approach views injury-prevention measures as positive, easy steps that enable people to continue enjoying life and taking risks.

To convey their message, SMARTRISK offers simple positive messages to navigate risk. The five key messages are:
- Buckle up.
- Look first.
- Wear the gear.
- Get trained.
- Drive sober.

These messages are applicable to all ages but are particularly appropriate for children, as it is important to influence beliefs at an early age. *Buckle up* is the message aimed at persuading people to make use of restraint devices whenever they are available. Whether in a car, an airplane, or a roller coaster, restraints reduce injury. To date, seat belts have saved more lives than any other intervention.[2] Proper use of child seats and booster seats can reduce infant deaths in car crashes by 71% and toddler deaths by 54%.[2] Children, however, are unlikely to be aware of the statistics and are unable to appreciate the consequences of not using seat belts. Therefore, injury prevention has to be targeted at parents as well. Parents need to understand that being good role models by wearing restraints consistently will have a much greater influence on the child's behaviour than anything they say to the child.[23] When a parent puts a helmet on a child but does not wear one himself, what message does that send? It sends a very strong message to the child that not wearing a helmet is a sign of maturity—and all children aspire to be perceived as mature.

*Look first* may refer to many things, including looking for traffic before crossing the road, checking the depth of the lake before diving in headfirst, looking over the crest of an unfamiliar ski hill before making a jump, or performing a circle check on the vehicle before driving.

*Wear the gear* applies to a wide variety of sporting or work-related activities. It might include wearing a helmet, wrist guards, and knee pads before taking to the streets on roller blades. It may refer to wearing PPE, such as gloves, goggles, and a mask, on paramedic calls.

*Get trained* may refer to driver training, WHMIS training, scuba diving lessons, family training in fire escape techniques, parent education on how to properly store household poisons, ski lessons, wilderness survival, or first-aid training.

*Drive sober* might also be called *drive without being impaired*. Impairment comes in many forms: alcohol impairment, drug impairment, emotional impairment (e.g., being angry or upset), sleep deprivation, or distraction (e.g., using a cellular phone, eating, or text messaging while driving). Driving requires full concentration. Incidents happen in a split second, and distractions of any kind have led to serious injury and death.

The question now is, how do we influence change in a positive way? How do we get to the heart of what matters most to people to make long-lasting change?

*Social Marketing.* Positive messages in injury prevention are the most influential and have the greatest long-term effect.[24,25] Social marketing, which is founded on the premise that positive messages result in positive outcomes, is aimed simply not at disseminating information, good or bad, about a product or service but at understanding the consumer's true needs and desires. This is what commercial marketers try to do. Once they understand the consumer's true needs and desires, the next step is to link their product or service to those needs and desires. For example, a television commercial depicts a university student studying abroad. The student laments that he misses the creature comforts of home back in Canada. In response, a certain coffee franchise sends him a case of his favourite coffee. The scene shows a glimpse into the student's thoughts: how the coffee brand reminds him of home, of his family and his friends, and of the time they spent sharing conversations over coffee. A link has now been established between the coffee brand and the student's needs and desires. Consumers watching the commercial relate to the student's longing for home, family, and friends and to the comfort associated with drinking the advertised coffee brand. It is a brilliant and effective marketing strategy.

Philip Kotler and Gerald Zaltman adapted basic marketing principles to create the science of social marketing to sell ideas, attitudes, and behaviours. Social marketing "has been used extensively in international health programs, especially for contraceptives and oral rehydration therapy (ORT), and is being used with more frequency in the United States for such diverse topics as drug abuse, heart disease and organ donation."[26]

Social marketing can also be applied to injury prevention. The objective is to learn what people want and need rather than trying to sell them what they *should* want or need. As injury-prevention advocates, we want to sell the public on the benefits of buckling up, looking first, wearing the gear, getting trained, and driving sober. Although these things may seem intuitively important to us, they do not have the same degree of importance for all people. Social marketers ask: *What is important to those people? How can we make the link between what is important and injury-prevention tenets?*

Consider the following true story. In a large warehouse located somewhere in Canada, the number of work-related injuries was high. Members of the occupational health and safety team had tried for many months to get employees to adhere to safety measures, including wearing hard hats and other PPE properly. Posters on safety equipment had been placed strategically. Supervisors regularly reminded staff to be careful in their work and to wear equipment as instructed. However, the number of injuries and the number of days lost to work-related injuries continued to rise. In frustration, the warehouse manager contacted SMARTRISK. A small team of injury-prevention experts came to the warehouse and began by getting an overview of the situation from the management. Soon after, they met with the workers one by one to get to know a little bit about them on a personal level. They asked less about their safety habits than about what was important to them in life and what they liked to do on their own time.

The team then went to the local school to meet the workers' children and grandchildren. They asked the children what they liked about their parents or grandparents and what they liked to do for fun with their family. While at the school, the team coordinated with teachers to have the children draw pictures of themselves playing with their parents and grandparents.

Again, the injury-prevention team met with the managers of the warehouse and discussed some injury-prevention strategies. A couple of days later, the team assembled all the workers in a large hall and put on a multimedia presentation. Set to music, which is known to influence our emotions, the presentation showed the workers' children and grandchildren. A 6-year-old boy, wearing a hard hat, said that he wanted his daddy to be safe so that they could play together forever and ever. A 5-year-old girl proudly showed a big card that she had made with a picture of her grandmother wearing gloves. The card read: "I need your hands to hold me. Love, Emily." The employees watched with great intensity, smiling, laughing, and crying. By the end of the presentation, there was not a dry eye in the room. The employees had seen the importance of safety through the eyes of their children and grandchildren. It gave them a new and fresh perspective on what before had been only a set of rules.

Social marketing goes to the heart of what is important to people and taps into the deeper reasons why safety is important. It strives to change the way people perceive risk from negative reinforcement to positive reinforcement.

*Harnessing the Power of the Media.* The media play an important role in influencing perception and behaviour. A University of Toronto study examined 250 automobile commercials and found that unsafe driving, including aggressive driving with speed violations, was evident in 25% of all commercials reviewed.[27] In contrast, safety was promoted in only 12% of the commercials studied.[27]

Injury-prevention organizations, public health departments, worker compensation boards, governments, and private industry have all used the media to promote injury-prevention messages. The cost of public service announcements on radio, television, billboards, and Web sites pales in comparison to the cost of injury, disability, and death due to injury.

Promoters of injury prevention can encourage the media to champion their cause by making changes as simple as incorporating the consistent use of seat belts in television shows, movies, and commercials. When depicting athletes or sporting events, advertising in any form, be it television or print media, can change the way the public perceives risks by ensuring the actors are wearing appropriate safety gear. By contacting local radio stations and requesting that announcers replace the word *accident* with *collision* or *crash* when broadcasting the traffic report, injury-prevention organizations can help change public perception.

The media are frequently eager to help reduce injury. Since virtually all radio stations are obliged to provide free air time for public service announcements, radio exposure is relatively inexpensive. The organization needs to prepare a well-thought-out message, to design and implement a plan that spans a specific period of time and to establish a means of measuring the outcome of the campaign.

## ENFORCEMENT

Enforcement—compelling people by law to change their behaviour—is a critical component of injury prevention.

Injury-prevention organizations should always include local, provincial or territorial, and federal law enforcement agencies in their stakeholder meetings and strategic planning. The police lend not only their expertise in law but also their experience as emergency responders to injuries of all kinds. They provide a unique perspective on injury prevention.

The power of the law to reduce injuries is well documented. In France, for example, the rate of traffic-related injuries was among the highest of all the European countries until 2002.[28] By doubling the number of police officers on the roads, focusing on drug- and alcohol-impaired drivers, and enforcing seat-belt use, the French police force were able to reduce the number of fatalities by 21% in a single year.[28]

After Korea doubled the penalty for not using safety restraints and mounted a well-publicized national police enforcement campaign, the use of seat belts rose from 23% to 98% in less than a year.[2]

In several Canadian provinces, compliance with seat-belt laws increased by 10–15% within one year of implementing similar high-profile enforcement programs.[2]

In contrast, laws regulating helmet use for cyclists are very difficult to enforce as cyclists may not carry identification documents with them, and in the case of children, the police have to contact parents when children break the law. Consequently, helmet use relies heavily on an honour system. Police, paramedics, public health departments, and other stakeholders need to join forces to create more innovative ways of increasing helmet use. One example that combines enforcement with innovation is the Please Be Seated car seat safety campaign in Peel Region, Ontario. In this program, a driver caught with an improperly installed car seat receives a fine and two demerit points. However, both the fine and the demerit points are waived if the driver attends a free car-seat education session by the Peel Car Seat Safety Committee.[29] The volunteer trainers include police officers, public health nurses, paramedics, and firefighters. Since as many as 80% of car seats are used incorrectly, this is an important injury-prevention issue.[30]

## ENGINEERING

Engineering refers to the creation and design of products or to changes to the environment to reduce injuries. Examples of injury-reducing design are abundant in all industries and include seat belts and air bags, needleless injection systems, sprinkler systems, bicycle training wheels, and grass medians on roads.

The benefit of injury prevention by design is that it is a passive countermeasure and requires little to no effort to change behaviour on the part of the consumer. Much as the passive countermeasure of immunization reduces the incidence of disease, engineering has proved to be the most effective form of injury prevention. However, many advances in engineering require accompanying education, behavioural, and enforcement components. Helmets may be brilliantly designed to protect the head, but children need to be persuaded to wear the helmets, and consistent, comprehensive laws should be enforced. Air bags are one of the greatest engineering feats of the past century, but drivers need to be persuaded to reduce their speed, keep a safe distance from other vehicles, make safe and appropriate lane changes, and drive free of hand-held distractions, and police need the necessary resources to enforce the laws.

Society often—arguably too often—relies on engineering to solve injury-causing issues. Either coincidentally or by consequence, technological advances have always outpaced the ability to change the way people perceive and respond to risk.[31] Of the traditional three Es, behaviour change through education is probably the most complex and challenging. Behaviour change, unlike engineering, is an active approach that requires people to recognize risk and take responsibility for protecting themselves and others. For this reason, the future of injury prevention will require the input not only of traditional stakeholders such as healthcare professionals, teachers, law officers, and engineers but also of behavioural science experts, who can address the fundamental issue of human perception.[31]

Injury-prevention campaigns must meet four criteria:
- Information about the risk must be comprehensive, straightforward, and honest.
- Persuasive messages must appeal to emotions.
- Training must be practical, with realistic steps.
- Feedback or enforcement must be as positive as possible.

## PARAMEDIC INVOLVEMENT IN INJURY PREVENTION

There are approximately 18,000 paramedics in Canada.[32] We are a small but highly skilled and specialized group who offer unique experience and insight to the injury-prevention field. Not only do paramedics have firsthand, intimate knowledge of *how* injuries happen, but we also go into homes, businesses, playing fields, farms, industrial complexes, and all other conceivable places *where* injuries happen. While statisticians collect data on mechanisms of injury, paramedics provide much of the eye-witness reporting of those mechanisms.

Paramedics make ideal ambassadors for injury prevention. However, we have to be wary about using negative reinforcement to deliver the injury-prevention message. As front-line responders, we see tragedy in its rawest form, and these disturbing images frequently inspire paramedics to play an active role in reducing injuries. Unfortunately, the haunting images that make us passionate and drive us to change our behaviour are only stories to the listening and viewing audiences who attend our impassioned lectures. They may be shocked and disturbed by the stories and images we have to share, but this does not translate into a change in behaviour on their part.[31] To bring about lasting change in behaviour, the emotional response to performing the behaviour must be more positive than negative.[33,34]

The following points support paramedic involvement in injury prevention:[7]
- Paramedics are often the most medically educated individuals in rural and remote settings.
- Paramedics are high-profile role models.
- Paramedics are often considered the champion of the customer.
- Paramedics are welcomed into homes, schools, and other environments.
- Paramedics are perceived by the public as authorities on injury and prevention.
- Paramedics are often the first to identify situations that pose a risk for illness or injury (e.g., unsanitary conditions, unsafe home environments).

## Protecting the Paramedic from Injury and Disease

Injury prevention should begin in-house. Making a contribution to reducing injury in the community is a noble pursuit, but it should occur in tandem with reducing injury risk in the paramedic field.

Although no Canadian statistics are available, it is likely that MVCs are a major cause of LODD, as they are in the United States.[12] In any case, driving is a large part of what paramedics do and should be the focus of internal injury-prevention strategies.

Other causes of injury, illness, and disability in paramedic practice include:
- Lifting
- Falls
- Needlestick/sharps
- Communicable disease transmission
- Chemical exposure
- Calls involving violence

## Educating the Educator

Paramedics need to become informed of the key issues in injury prevention, both those in which they can have a positive influence and those over which they have less control. Next, paramedics need to seek out other injury-prevention organizations to learn from their collective experience and wisdom. Are there paramedics currently working with injury-prevention organizations in your area? What is their role?

## Leading by Example

Paramedics are highly influential role models to their community and to their family and friends, whether they are aware of it or not. As role models, they have an obligation to be informed and to practise safety routinely. For example, people should see that paramedics wear their seat belts at all times, whether in an ambulance or while driving their personal cars. In social settings, friends should see that paramedics drive sober and that they do not allow friends or family members to drive impaired. Paramedics who *look first* before diving into water, *wear the gear* when snowboarding, boating, or cycling, and practise other forms of injury prevention in their own daily lives send a powerful message to the public that these steps reduce risks and save lives.

## Research and Injury Prevention

While it is admirable to be passionate about injury prevention, it is critical that we seek out tangible results so that we *know* that our activities have a positive and measurable result. Personal conviction is not sufficient; our energies are better spent in activities that make a difference. This is the role that research plays in injury prevention.

The objective is to reduce injuries. The question is how? What works? To answer this question requires a two-fold approach. First, we need to track injury through surveillance. This involves keeping provincial, territorial, and national databases that include patient age, location, time of day, type of injury, mechanism of injury, and any other epidemiological information that might shed light on causes and prevention strategies. Second, research programs need to be adequately funded to address the issue. Although injuries account for 11% all healthcare costs in Canada, less than 1% of all available research funds are directed toward its prevention.[35]

Injury-prevention partners from across Canada have recommended the following goals:[36]

▓  Establish a strategic injury research agenda focused on areas where injury reduction would produce the greatest health, social, and economic gains.
▓  Partner with the Canadian Institutes of Health Research (CIHR) to co-fund team development grants.
▓  Establish an Injury Research and Demonstration Fund to test and evaluate approaches to injury prevention and control.
▓  Create a National Injury Information and Education Committee comprising all major stakeholders to coordinate the translation and dissemination of injury research findings and incorporate them into information and activities in the field.

## Paramedic Data Collection

Paramedics play a critical role in the process of collecting injury data. The information you ascertain from the scene about patient age, location, time of injury, injury type and severity, neurological status, vital signs, and mechanism of injury is all essential to **injury surveillance** databases. Patient demographic documentation is also critical for tracking purposes. Information such as first and last names, date of birth, and health card number can all be used in the future for retrieval of important out-of-hospital information. The more information that the paramedic can collect on how the injury happened, the more useful it is to the injury-prevention programmer. Charting that someone fell while trying to get out of bed or while walking down the stairs is more helpful than simply stating that the patient fell.

## Support and Resources for Injury-Prevention Activities

Fire and police services have a long history of injury prevention. In fact, most urban fire and police services have staff, and in some cases whole departments, dedicated to this function. Paramedic services are comparatively new to the injury-prevention forum, and therefore most services must organize and lobby for local, provincial, or territorial funding. To convince the public and politicians of the need for paramedic involvement, a significant amount of volunteerism is required. Money does not flow freely into proposed new programs unless it can be demonstrated that those seeking it are uniquely qualified, can contribute in a meaningful and measurable way, and have a high level of interest and goodwill.

## Empowering Individual Paramedics to Conduct Primary Injury Prevention

Paramedics can demonstrate the importance of their participation in injury prevention through individual volunteering. By participating in existing injury-prevention organizations, paramedics can begin to establish both themselves and the profession as an essential resource.

## Activities

There are many organizations across Canada that paramedics can join to assist in injury-prevention activities (see Box 2-2). If your service is not yet involved directly in injury-prevention activities, there are many organizations to choose from.

One such program is Prevent Alcohol and Risk-Related Trauma in Youth (PARTY), a hospital-hosted interactive injury prevention and health-promotion program for teenagers. There are over 60 PARTY program sites across Canada and the United States. This program was founded because the greatest incidence of death and injury occurs in the 15–24 year age group. It was created to educate teens on the perils of risk-taking behaviour and the tragic consequences that can occur.

In a full-day session, students follow the path of an injury survivor, meeting the professionals, including paramedics, who would care for the survivor. Various health professionals describe the journey of a trauma patient and present facts about head and spinal cord injury. The students get hands-on experience with the equipment used in trauma care and rehabilitation. What separates this program from other "reality" programs is that it is interactive, no one lectures the students on what *not* to do, and the messages, although sometimes disturbing, are positive. Students get a first-hand glimpse into the reality of injury and are given choices—the choices that will help them live well and live long. The most powerful part of the day is the injury survivor presentation. Students meet and talk with young injury survivors who speak frankly about their

| BOX 2–2 | Canadian Organizations Involved in Injury Prevention |
|---|---|

Atlantic Network for Injury Prevention
http://www.anip.ca

Alberta Health and Wellness
http://www.health.gov.ab.ca

Alberta Centre for Injury Control and Research
http://www.med.ualberta.ca/acicr

British Columbia Injury Research and Prevention Unit
http://www.injuryresearch.bc.ca

Canadian Agricultural Safety Association
http://www.casa-acsa.ca

Canadian Agricultural Surveillance Program
http://meds.queensu.ca/~emresrch/caisp/
http://www.meds.queensu.ca/-emresrch/~

Canadian Association of Fire Chiefs
http://www.cafc.ca

Canadian Automobile Association
http://www.caa.ca

Canadian Centre for Occupational Health and Safety
http://www.ccohs.ca

Canadian Firearms Centre
http://www.cfc-ccaf.gc.ca

Canadian Health Network
http://www.canadian-health-network.ca

Canadian Injury Prevention and Control Curriculum
http://www.canadianinjurycurriculum.ca

Canadian Institute of Child Health
http://www.cich.ca

Canadian Paediatric Society
http://www.cps.ca

Canadian Public Health Association
http://www.cpha.ca

Canadian Red Cross
http://www.redcross.ca

Canadian Road Safety Professionals
http://www.carpsp.ca

Canadians for Responsible and Safe Highways
http://www.web.net/~crash

Canadian Injury Research Network
http://www.cirnet.ca

Canadian Institutes of Health Research
http://www.cihr-irsc.gc.ca/index.html

Canadian Institutes for Health Information
http://www.cihr-irsc.gc.ca

Canada Safety Council
http://www.safety-council.org

Centre for Surveillance Coordination, Public Health Agency
of Canada
http://www.phac-aspc.gc.ca/surveillance_e.html
http://www.phac-aspc.gc.ca

Child Safety Link
http://www.childsafetylink.ca

Health Canada
http://www.hc-sc.gc.ca

Insurance Bureau of Canada
http://www.ibc.ca

IMPACT, Injury Prevention Centre of Children's Hospital
http://www.hsc.mb.ca/impact/

KIDSAFE Connection, Stolley Children's Health Centre
http://www.capitalhealth.ca

Lifesaving Society
http://www.lifesaving.ca

Mothers Against Drunk Driving
http://www.madd.ca

National Clearinghouse on Family Violence
http://www.phac-aspc.gc.ca/ncfv-cnivf/familyviolence/

Nova Scotia Health Promotion and Protection
http://www.gov.ns.ca/hpp

Prevent Alcohol and Risk Related Trauma in Youth (PARTY)
Program
http://www.partyprogram.com

Plan-It Safe, Children's Hospital of Eastern Ontario
http://www.plan-itsafe.com

Quebec WHO Collaborating Centre for Safety Promotion
and Injury Prevention
http://www.inspq.qc.ca/ccOMS/SecuriteTrauma/

Quebec Public Health
http://www.inspq.qc.ca

Rick Hansen Foundation
http://www.rickhansen.com

Safe Communities Foundation
http://www.safecommunities.ca

Safe Kids Canada
http://www.sickkids.ca/safekidscanada/

Safe Start
http://www.bcchildrens.ca/KidsTeensFam/ChildSafety/SafeStart/
default.htm

SMARTRISK
http://www.smartrisk.ca

Saskatchewan Institute on Prevention of Handicaps
http://www.PreventionInstitute.sk.ca

St. John Ambulance
http://www.sja.ca

ThinkFirst Foundation
http://www.thinkfirst.ca

Transport Canada Transportation Safety
http://www.tc.gc.ca

injuries, the events that led to them, and what their lives are like now.

Many of the public health units and government agencies across Canada offer, or are affiliated with organizations that offer, car seat safety inspection programs. The Canada Safety Council, in partnership with private industry, for example, offers the Buckle Up Bears Care Seat Program. Paramedics can attend workshops to learn to inspect car seats for infants, toddlers, and small children and to advise parents on properly securing their children.

According to first-aid agencies, the personal injury rate is reduced by as much as 40% among participants who have been trained in first aid.[37,38] Since many paramedics already teach first aid, this is a simple, accessible, and practical way for paramedics to have an effect on injury reduction.

There are numerous opportunities for paramedics to play an active role in injury-prevention initiatives. A brief search for programs in your area should include the public health department, local hospitals, and emergency services.

## Implementation and Prevention Strategies

A report published by SMARTRISK, *Ending Canada's Invisible Epidemic: A Strategy for Injury Prevention*, aims to reduce Canada's injury rate to the lowest of any country in the world.[36] To accomplish this, the report calls on the government of Canada to develop a National Injury Prevention Strategy with the following six pillars:

1. National leadership and coordination
   * Establish an Injury Prevention Centre of Canada (IPCC) as part of the new Public Health Agency of Canada.
   * Give IPCC a distinct budget and mandate to promote evidence-based strategies for injury prevention.
2. An effective surveillance system
   * Establish a National Injury Surveillance Coordinating Committee (NISCC) within the IPCC to monitor injury trends and issue an annual report.
3. Research
   * The IPCC should build a cadre of injury researchers and foster the translation of knowledge into action.
4. Community supports and resources
   * Establish a National Injury Prevention Community Fund and a clearinghouse, maintained by the IPCC, to provide communities with financial resources, information, and tools to implement evidence-based injury-prevention strategies and to share information.
5. Policy analysis and development
   * The IPCC should provide governments with expert information and analysis and help facilitate the introduction of evidence-based policies, regulations, and programs to reduce the risk for injury in Canada.
   * Activities would include regular scans of international policy to pinpoint new evidence and effective practices and reviews of domestic policies to identify opportunities for action.
6. Public information and education
   * The IPCC should develop communication strategies to support national injury-prevention targets and goals.
   * Strategies should include marketing campaigns, media relations, and the development of reference materials.

## HEALTH PROMOTION

The Government of Canada recognizes that many diseases are linked to lifestyle choices and acknowledges that there "are enormous potential benefits to be derived from health and wellness promotion".[39] The first step is to determine which diseases pose the greatest healthcare risks and which ones can be affected by and changed through health promotion.

Cardiovascular disease is the number-one cause of death in Canada. Consequently, education in the field of lifestyle change or risk factor modification is one of the key objectives of the Heart and Stroke Foundation of Canada (HSFC). The HSFC describes a chain of survival to increase the chances of survival from a heart attack or stroke. The chain has seven links:

1. Healthy choices to reduce risks of heart attack and stroke.
2. Early recognition of the signs and symptoms of heart attack and stroke.
3. Early access through 911 or a local emergency number.
4. Early CPR.
5. Early defibrillation.
6. Early advanced care.
7. Early rehabilitation.

Paramedics are educated in the knowledge and skills best suited for links 4 through 6: CPR, defibrillation, and advanced care. Paramedics can also help with links 1 and 2 by instructing CPR classes, speaking to special-interest groups, and taking other opportunities to educate the public about healthy choices and the early recognition of the signs and symptoms of heart attack and stroke. Because many heart attacks and strokes occur in the home and are witnessed by family members, who often are untrained, educating high school students in CPR will help improve the chances of survival. Some provincial ministries of education have implemented mandatory CPR training for high school students, and in many schools where mandatory CPR does not exist, CPR training is provided on a volunteer basis. Paramedics can lend their support to teachers and schools to facilitate these programs (see ACT Foundation Weblink, Chapter 1).

## Health Screening

A large part of public health deals with screening the public for early signs of heart disease, diabetes, or other health problems. This is also an area in which many paramedic services are involved. Screening might include assessment of blood pressure for early detection of hypertension and assessment of blood sugar for early detection of diabetes or assessment of medication compliance.

## Immunization Programs

More and more paramedics are joining forces with their local public health departments to assist in providing immunizations or flu shots at public clinics during the fall and winter. With the provinces and territories actively promoting flu vaccination for all Canadians, public health nurses and hospitals are challenged to meet the demand. This is both an important community service and an active means of health promotion.

## Paramedic Practice and Community Health

The following list of community health initiatives in which Nova Scotia paramedics are involved is an example of the expanded scope of practice that paramedics can expect to see in the future:

- Congestive heart failure assessment
- Fall prevention and home safety assessment
- Venipuncture and phlebotomies
- Urinalysis
- Removal of sutures and staples
- Wound care
- Immunizations
- Medication compliance
- Diabetic assessment
- Glucose checks
- Blood pressure checks
- Antibiotic administration
- $B_{12}$ injections
- Helmet safety fitting
- Car-seat installation
- CPR and first-aid instruction
- Health promotion activities

# SUMMARY

- Worldwide, injury is the leading cause of death and disability between birth and age 59. In Canada, injuries are the leading cause of death for those aged 1 to 44.
- The cost to the Canadian economy due to unintentional injuries alone is estimated at $8.7 billion annually.
- Paramedics need to be aware of injury risk within their own profession. For example, motor vehicle collisions (MVCs) are the leading cause of line-of-duty death (LODD) for paramedics.
- Injury is predictable and preventable.
- Prevention begins with an acknowledgment that injury is one of Canada's most serious and most expensive healthcare problems.
- The three Es of injury prevention are Education, Enforcement (law), and Engineering.
- Positive education achieves more than scare tactics. Social marketing has proven to be very effective.
- Research is essential to ensure that activities have a positive and measurable result.
- Paramedics are playing an active role in injury prevention throughout Canada.
- Some ambulance services have sought and received funding to support injury-prevention activities, while others rely on volunteerism and partnerships with organizations with similar goals.
- Paramedic associations also play a large role in promoting injury prevention. Paramedics are a valuable resource in the public health domain.
- Paramedics are involved in health screening of the general public for early signs of heart disease, diabetes, or other health problems.
- Immunization is another area of health promotion where paramedics can join forces with their local public health departments.

# WEBLINKS

- SMARTRISK: This leading national nonprofit injury-prevention organization enjoys international recognition and support. SMARTRISK also works closely and extensively with other injury-prevention organizations across Canada.
  http://www.smartrisk.ca
- The Cochrane Collaboration: This international not-for-profit organization produces and disseminates systematic reviews of healthcare interventions and promotes the search for evidence. The Web site offers an extensive review of injury-prevention research.
  www.cochrane.org

## ● ● ● REFERENCES

1. Peden M, McGee K, Krug E, eds. *Injury 2000: A Leading Cause of the Global Burden of Disease.* World Health Organization; 2002, p.7.

2. Peden M, Scurfield R, Sleet D, et al., eds. *World Report on Road Traffic Injury Prevention: Summary.* World Health Organization; 2004, p.16.

3. Ottawa Safe Communities Network: *Who Is Injured?* 2000. Available at: http://www.ottawasafecommunities.org/statistics.htm. Accessed July 18, 2006.

4. Statistics Canada, Health Statistics Division. *Selected Leading Causes of Death, by Sex. Age-standardized mortality rate per 100,000 population.* Last modified: 2005-02-17. Available at: http://www40.statcan.ca/l01/cst01/health36.htm. Accessed July 18, 2006.

5. Health Canada. *Injuries.* Available at: http://www.statcan.ca/english/freepub/82-221-XIE/01002/high/region/hinjuries.htm. Accessed July 18, 2006.

6. Angus DE,, Cloutier JE, Albert T, Chénard D, Shariatmader A. *The Economic Burden of Unintentional Injury in Canada.* SMARTRISK Foundation; 1998.

7. Sanders MJ. *Mosby's Paramedic Textbook,* 3rd ed. St. Louis, MO: Mosby; 2005.

8. Canadian Institute for Health Information, National Trauma Registry: *Causes of Injury Admissions in Children (<20 years), Canada, 1999/2000.* Available at: http://secure.cihi.ca/cihiweb/dispPage.jsp?cw_page=home_e. Accessed July 18, 2006.

9. Public Health Agency of Canada. *The Economic Burden of Unintentional Injury in Canada,* 1998. Available at: http://www.phac-aspc.gc.ca/injury-bles/ebuic-febnc/index.html. Accessed July 18, 2006.

10. Health Canada and Transport Canada Injury Surveillance Program and The Road Safety Program. *Road Safety in Canada: An Overview.* 2004.

11. Canadian Institute for Health Information (CIHI), Ontario Trauma Registry. *Injury Hospitalizations in Ontario.* 2004.

12. Maguire BJ, Hunting KL, Smith GS, Levick NR. Occupational fatalities in emergency medical services: A hidden crisis. *Ann Emerg Med.* 2002;40:6.

13. Blahey GG. *Canadian Occupational Safety: Farmers wait for the health and safety system to address their unique concerns.* 2003. Available at: http://www.industrialsourcebook.com/cgi-bin/archivecos.pl?id=561. Accessed July 19, 2006.

14. Canadian Safety Council. *What to Teach Your Children About Bicycle Safety.* 2005. Available at: http://www.safety-council.org/info/child/bicycle.htm. Accessed July 19, 2006.

15. Canadian Red Cross. *What We Have Learned: 10 Years of Pertinent Facts About Drownings and Other Water-Related Injuries in Canada, 1991–2000.*

16. Canadian Institute for Health Information. *Recreational Injuries: Summary Statistics for Sports and Recreational Activities Resulting in Severe Injuries, by Type, 2000/2001.* Available at: http://secure.cihi.ca/cihiweb/en/media_15jan2003_tab1_e.html, Accessed July 19, 2006.

17. Canadian Institute for Health Information. *Most Snowmobile-Related Injuries Occur in February: Youth are the most likely to sustain serious snowmobile-related injuries.* Available at:

http://www.cihi.ca/cihiweb/dispPage.jsp?cw_page=media_25jan2006_e. Accessed July 19, 2006.

18. World Health Organization. *World Report on Road Traffic Injury Prevention, 2004.* Available at: http://www.who.int/violence_injury_prevention. Accessed July 19, 2006.

19. Canada Safety Council. *Higher Speeds Drive Traffic Deaths Up: Fast Driving is an Emerging Safety Problem.* 2006. Available at: http://www.safety-council.org/info/traffic/speed.html. Accessed July 19, 2006.

20. Haddon W. Options for the prevention of motor vehicle crash injury. *Isr J Med Sci.*1980;16:45–65.

21. Canadian Hospitals Injury Reporting and Prevention Program (CHIRPP), Public Health Agency of Canada. *Data Sampler: Injuries Associated With Playground Equipment.* 2000. Available at: www.phac-aspc.gc.ca/injury-bles/. Accessed July 19, 2006.

22. Canadian Centre for Occupational Health and Safety (CCOHS), Association of Workers' Compensation Boards of Canada, Workplace Health, Safety and Compensation Commission of New Brunswick, eds. *Influencing Attitudes Towards Workplace Illnesses and Injuries.* Hamilton, Ont: CCOHS; 1998.

23. Research Coordination Unit, Queen's University. *Better Beginnings, Better Futures: A Comprehensive Community Based Early Childhood Development Project.* 2006. Available at: http://bonpas.queensu.ca/pub.html. Accessed July 19, 2006.

24. Geller ES. A behavioral science approach to transportation safety. *Bull NY Acad Med.* 1988; 632.

25. Geller ES, Kalsher MJ, Rudd JR, Lehman GR. Promoting safety belt use on a university campus: An integration of commitment and incentive strategies. *J Appl Soc Psych.* 1989; 19: 3–19.

26. Kline WN. *What Is Social Marketing?* 2003. Available at: www.social-marketing.com. Accessed July 19, 2006.

27. Shin PC, Hallett D, Chipman ML, Tator C, Granton JT. Unsafe driving in North American automobile commercials. *J Public Health Med.* 2005; 27(4): 318–325.

28. SMARTRISK. *Crash Rate Down in France.* Available at: http://www.smartrisk.ca/ContentDirector.aspx?tp=1064&dd=8. Accessed July 19, 2006.

29. Region of Peel. News Release. *Child Car Seat Inspection Program Huge Success.* 2000. Available at: http://www.region.peel.on.ca/news/archiveitem.asp?year=2001&month=10&day=26&file=20011026a.xml. Accessed July 19, 2006.

30. Ontario Ministry of Transportation. *Love Me Buckle Me Right.* 2004. Available at: http://ogov.newswire.ca/ontario/GPOE/2004/04/16/c1708.html?lmatch=&lang=_e.html. Accessed July 19, 2006.

31. Carlson Gielen A, Sleet D. Application of behavior-change theories and methods to injury prevention. *Epidemiol Rev.* 2003;25:65–76.

32. 37th Parliament, 2nd Session, Standing Committee on Finance. *Number of Paramedics in Canada. 1435 hours.* 2003. Available at: http://www.parl.gc.ca/committee/CommitteePublication.aspx?SourceId=66790. Accessed July 19, 2006.

33. Fishbein M. Developing effective behavior change interventions: Some lessons learned from behavioral research. In: Backer TE, David SL, Soucy G, eds. *Reviewing the Behavioral*

*Science Knowledge Base on Technology Transfer.* Bethesda, MD: National Institute on Drug Abuse, 1995. NIDA Research Monograph, no. 155.

34. Fishbein M, Triandis HC, Kanfer FH, et al. Factors influencing behavior and behavior change. In: Baum A, Tevenson TA, Singer JE, eds. *Handbook of Health Psychology.* Mahwah, NJ: Lawrence Erlbaum Associates; 2001.

35. Cusimano MD, Mukhida K. *Acute Injuries Research in Canada: Background Paper for the Canadian Institute for Health Research Listening for Direction in Injury.* 2003. Available at: http://www.injurypreventionstrategy.ca/ downloads/LFDI_Acute.pdf. Accessed July 19, 1006.

36. SMARTRISK. *Ending Canada's Invisible Epidemic: A Strategy for Injury Prevention,* 2005.

37. Red Cross. *Preventing Injury and Drowning.* Available at: http://www.redcross.ca/article.asp?id=003039&tid=085. Accessed July 19, 2006.

38. St. John Ambulance. *Injury Rate Reduced.* Available at: http://stjohnambulance.ns.ca/index.php?menid= 02&mtyp=1. Accessed July 19, 2006.

39. Government of Canada. *The Health of Canadian: The Federal Role.* 2002. Available at: http://www.parl.gc.ca/37/2/parlbus/ commbus/senate/com-e/SOCI-E/rep-e/repoct02vol6part5-e. htm. Accessed July 19, 2006.

# CHAPTER 3

# Medical–Legal Aspects of Paramedic Practice

## ● ● ● OBJECTIVES

*Upon completion of this chapter, the paramedic student will be able to:*

1. Describe the basic structure of the legal system in Canada.
2. Relate how laws affect the paramedic's practice, including transportation.
3. List situations for the paramedic that are subject to statutory reporting in most provinces and territories.
4. Describe the four elements involved in a claim of negligence.
5. Describe measures paramedics may take to protect themselves from claims of negligence.
6. Describe the paramedic's responsibilities with regard to patient confidentiality.
7. Describe and contrast the various forms of consent and outline the process for obtaining consent.
8. Describe legal complications relating to consent.

9. Describe actions to be taken in a refusal-of-care situation.
10. Describe legal considerations related to patient transportation.
11. Outline legal issues related to specific resuscitation situations.
12. List and describe the actions to be taken in a refusal-of-care situation to guard from legal action.
13. List measures the paramedic should take to preserve evidence when responding to a death, crime, or accident scene.
14. Detail the components of effective legal reports and documentation of medical information.
15. Define common medical-legal terms that apply to prehospital situations involving patient care.

## ● ● ● KEY TERMS

## THE LEGAL AND ETHICAL FRAMEWORK FOR PARAMEDIC PRACTICE

The Paramedic has legal obligations to the patient, the employer, the public at large and, where applicable, to the governing structure of the EMS system in place in a given province or territory. These obligations give rise to expec- tations and exposures, or risks, to the paramedic, and form the legal framework within which the paramedic will prac- tice at all times. Superimposed on the legal framework are the expectations of the public to fair, accessible, and nondiscriminatory care by knowledgeable, skilled, and car- ing individuals trained in the emergency care of ill, injured, and incapacitated individuals. That forms the basis for the ethical framework within which the paramedic works.

## Sources of Law in Canada

There are two main sources of law in Canada: statute and common law. Statute is generally legislated and enacted by the federal, provincial, or territorial governments. Some lesser authority to legislate may be delegated to municipalities and regions, but that rarely results in significant legal risk or exposure for a paramedic.

The Canadian Constitution sets out the division of powers, or jurisdiction, between the federal government and the provinces or territories of Canada. As an example, criminal law is the exclusive legislative jurisdiction of the federal government and applies across the country. Provinces have no ability to amend or refuse to apply those laws. Provinces have jurisdiction to enact laws that apply locally within the province, such as traffic laws, which may vary between or among the provinces or territories.

There may be shared or overlapping jurisdiction within defined limits. For instance, generally, provinces are responsible for human rights and workplace or employment-related laws, but the federal government retains and exercises the right to regulate federal industry and related workplaces, such as banking and transportation. As well, federal privacy or equity laws may apply provincially, within explicit limitations.

Except with respect to criminal conduct, the legal framework for paramedic practice is generally within the provincial jurisdiction, although coroner's inquests or public inquiries can be federal or provincial. Most, including civil law proceedings, are provincial or territorial.

### CIVIL LAW

The basis of civil law in all provinces and territories in Canada, except Quebec, is common law. Common law has its roots in the British legal system. It derives from the interpretation and application of legal principles to individual fact situations, based on the underlying premise that like circumstances should be judged similarly, having regard to considerations of law and equity. Law generally refers to statute; equity refers to principles of fairness that may determine an issue on other than pure legal grounds.

Common law is often referred to as "judge-made" law. The principles of common law flow from the grounds (or basis) in law for a decision that interprets or applies legal and equitable (fairness considerations that may modify a strict reading application of law or legislation) principles. That reasoning carries weight in future court decisions, with the weighting dependent on the hierarchical level of the court in which the decision is made. Most court proceedings start in lower provincial courts, moving up through higher provincial levels on appeal or referral, or ultimately to the Supreme Court of Canada. Once a decision is affirmed or concluded at the Supreme Court of Canada level, the decision affects all similar fact situations as the applicable principles of interpretation in like cases in all provinces and territories, and at all court levels. This is referred to as a precedent. For

instance, the legal test for **negligence** (i.e., that of the reasonable or prudent man having regard to all of the circumstances) is based on the legal reasoning in Donoghue v. Stevenson,* a case from the British House of Lords in 1932 that predates the recognition of the Supreme Court of Canada as Canada's highest court level.

Except for the Supreme Court of Canada, whose decisions are precedents throughout Canada, decisions at other court levels are precedents only for lower level court(s) within the applicable province or territory. However, even without establishing precedent, those decisions can affect other court rulings as the grounds, or reason, for a decision may be persuasive in another court or jurisdiction.

The only notable exception to the system of common law in Canada is in Quebec. Quebec civil law is premised on the French Civil Code, which has its roots in European Civil Law. It has a different basis for decision making that may not apply the same guiding principles. As a result, Quebec decisions, including those made at the Supreme Court of Canada level may have a limited precedential value in the rest of Canada, and decisions elsewhere in Canada may have limited effect in Quebec.

### PUBLIC AND PRIVATE LAW

Law in Canada may also be characterized generally as public or private law. Public law reflects the nature or source of disputes between the individual and the state, such as criminal, tax, environmental, labour, and regulatory laws, including the regulation of healthcare professionals. Provincial public law, which generally pertains to matters governing the health and welfare of individuals, are generally determined in accordance with common law principles in all jurisdictions, except Quebec, where the Quebec Civil Code applies.

Federal public law statutes, including the Criminal Code, narcotic drug laws, federal taxation laws, and Trade and Commerce and National Security laws, apply equally in all provinces and jurisdictions, although the administration and enforcement of these laws may be the responsibility of, or shared with, the provinces. Accordingly, the application of common law doctrines and principles in these areas will apply equally in Quebec as elsewhere.

Administrative law may be viewed as a subset of public law. It comprises statutes and regulations enacted to regulate specific organizations or activities for the protection or support of the general public. The Ambulance Act of Ontario and the Regulated Health Professions Act of Ontario are examples of administrative law. The first regulates ambulance service in the province; the second prescribes the regulation of healthcare professionals practising in the province.

Private law is the term applicable to disputes between two or more named individuals. Individuals may include

---

*[1932] A.C. 562 (H.L.) at p. 580

organizations or legal entities. Examples include employment, contract, tort, family, property, and estate laws. Most private law, or civil, disputes, including malpractice and negligence claims, are referred to as civil suits. They may give rise to civil liability, which is usually characterized by claims for monetary compensation. Other remedies, such as a directive to do or cease to do something, may also apply in exceptional circumstances.

In all instances of law, public or private, the governing legislative authority also has the authority to pass regulations to further interpret or clarify the main statute or to specify how the governing statute is to be applied and enforced.

## Scope and Standards of Practice

In addition to the formal legal framework within which a paramedic must practise, there are also formal and informal public expectations that will govern the scope and **standards of practice**. These responsibilities are shaped (and may be prescribed in part) by ethical considerations that apply in the exercise of professional judgment and day-to-day decision making in practice settings. Scope and standards of practice may include formally written (including legislated) or explicit duties and obligations and informal norms and customs that have virtually the same weight as if they were formally entrenched in law.

## EFFECT OF LAWS AND LEGAL ACCOUNTABILITY FOR THE PARAMEDIC

Paramedics must act in a manner, whether providing care or providing transportation to patients, that is consistent with their education and training, expected standards of practice, and legal requirements. A failure to fully live up to any one of these aspects, or even an allegation of such failure, may result in legal liability to the paramedic and to the EMS organization employing the paramedic.

In addition, paramedics are expected to maintain current knowledge and proficiency in the skills within their scope of practice and to behave morally and ethically in their duties. Because of the rapid changes in out-of-hospital care, paramedics are also expected to demonstrate a lifelong commitment to continuing medical education. They are expected to do these things to ensure that the public is protected under law from unreasonable risk of harm.

It is notable that an error in judgment does not necessarily constitute negligence and will not necessarily result in a finding of civil liability if it can be demonstrated, using testimony from peers within the same profession, with the same level of certification, similar experience, and standing, that under similar circumstances they might have made the same or similar error.

A failure to adhere to expected ethical and legal guidelines and requirements can result in exposure to legal risk and penalties for the paramedic. The typical areas of legal exposure or liability arise from employment, criminal, civil, and, if applicable, professional regulations and standards, or from exposure to coroners' proceedings. Penalties can include an order to pay monetary compensation, fines, discipline up to and including loss of employment and/or professional accreditation, incarceration (for criminal acts or omissions), and/or legal directives affecting the paramedic's continued scope of or ability to practise.

Penalties for deficient practice resulting in harm to a patient may include any combination of the foregoing and may result from more than one proceeding. For instance, criminal conduct resulting in harm to a patient or employer may result in a criminal prosecution, a civil suit, and an employment proceeding such as a grievance or wrongful dismissal suit. If the harm includes a death, the matter may also be the subject of a coroner's inquiry or inquest. Where applicable, a professional misconduct prosecution is also likely from the paramedic's governing regulatory body. If there are allegations of a breach of human rights in the fact situation in issue, there may also be a human rights challenge or inquiry.

## SOURCES OF LEGAL EXPOSURE AND LIABILITY

### Legal Exposure Through Employment and Employment Liability

The most common but least recognized source of legal exposure for a paramedic is with respect to employment-related matters. A paramedic as an employee is subject to a range of employment obligations and responsibilities in addition to professional expectations. Every employment relationship includes an implicit assumption that an employee will serve the employer's services faithfully and competently and will obey the lawful orders and directives of that employer. In exchange, the employee can rely on payment for those services, subject to lawful deductions. In addition, every workplace is subject to employment-related legislation that establishes minimum workplace standards, including occupational health and safety, human rights, employment standards, and others. For the paramedic, regulatory legislation may also impose additional responsibilities and expectations with respect to conduct, scope, and standards of practice. For instance, provincial or territorial highway traffic statutes usually have specific provisions applicable to emergency services.

In addressing the reciprocal responsibilities and obligations of the workplace, the paramedic can expect to meet a range of situations in which he or she may be involved. The paramedic is responsible to the employer for his or her own practice and conduct but may also have obligations with respect to the employer's interests and those of the public in recognizing and reporting others' serious misconduct or behaviour in the course of discharging their own duties and obligations (e.g., reporting of a drug error, assault of a patient or any serious misconduct by his/her partner). Employment–related issues, with resultant legal exposure, may include a human rights complaint, a workplace dispute, including workers' compensation or employment insurance claims, and issues with respect to competence, scope, and standards of practice.

Exposures and likelihood of involvement in employment-related legal proceedings increase if the paramedic is employed in a unionized workplace and if the paramedic is himself or herself a union member. Unionized workforces have access to workplace dispute resolution processes, including grievances and arbitration, and may be participants in legal job action in the course of contract negotiations. Even if the paramedic is not a union member, he or she may be impacted by such proceedings in the workplace as a witness or as a result of general workplace disruption resulting from labour relations considerations. For instance, a job sanction such as strike action by unionized workers in a hospital or in a location to which a paramedic is called may delay, disrupt, or impede the paramedic's response or treatment time but does not change the essential nature of the paramedic's obligations to the patient. For instance, the paramedic cannot refuse a call solely because there is a hospital picket line in place.

The paramedic may be involved as a witness or as a direct (named) participant. Employment-related legal exposure is sometimes in addition to other legal exposures such as a coroner's inquest or inquiry, a civil suit, or professional liability proceeding. Except with respect to a coroner's inquest or inquiry, the employee as witness will rarely incur employment liability, unless in the course of acting as a witness some previously unknown misconduct is discovered.

Employment liability is typically addressed by a range of disciplinary penalties, ranging from a verbal warning to an unpaid suspension or, in the case of serious misconduct or incompetence, to termination of employment. In addition, or in the alternative, performance concerns that do not constitute incompetence may result in remedies intended to address and correct the deficiencies. Often, these are addressed first in nondisciplinary ways but may result in disciplinary sanction where the employee fails to improve or to meet the required standard and expectations.

## Coroner's Inquests and Inquiries

Every jurisdiction in Canada has a legislated system, commonly known as a coroner's system, for investigation into sudden or suspicious deaths. Because of the nature of the paramedic's practice, he or she can reasonably expect to be involved in such investigations, whether or not the paramedic is aware of that involvement or not. As the first medical responder in most critical situations, the paramedic's notes and observations often inform the coroner of some of the initial or situational circumstances of the deceased. If the matter proceeds to inquest or inquiry, the paramedic may be summoned to a formal proceeding as a witness to give evidence under oath. Typically, the testimony relates to the initial circumstances of the deceased and of the care or treatment rendered at the scene and on transport, up to

and including the turnover to trained hospital personnel, if the deceased was alive or resuscitation efforts were initiated when first attended by the paramedic.

Every jurisdiction in Canada has mandatory reporting requirements, although the specifics vary between jurisdictions. Factors that generally are considered include

- death as a result of violence, accident, or suicide;
- poisoning;
- maternal death during or following pregnancy;
- death as a result of alleged inappropriate or negligent treatment;
- death on a construction or industrial site;
- death that occurs during or within a set period following administration of a general anaesthetic or invasive procedure; and
- any death that occurs unexpectedly, particularly where the deceased was believed to be in good health.

The legislation generally prescribes the persons/professionals obligated to report. Most often this can be done through the police, but reporting requirements and specifics can vary by jurisdiction, so the paramedic must be aware of the expectations and requirements in his or her practice area.

Very few coroners' cases proceed to inquest or inquiry. Usually, an investigation is conducted by the coroner or medical examiner with the assistance of the police. Most terminate after investigation. Where it is determined to be in the public interest, the coroner may decide to advance the matter to inquest or inquiry.

An inquest is an inquisitorial (as opposed to a criminal prosecution or civil law suit, which is adversarial) process that serves a fact-finding function to answer five questions about the circumstances of the death:

- Who was the deceased?
- When did the deceased die?
- Where did the deceased die?
- How did the deceased die?
- By what means did the deceased die?

The proceeding is formal, and witnesses are compelled to give evidence under oath. Provinces and territories differ with respect to who presides over the proceeding. Dependent on jurisdiction, it may be the coroner or a provincial/territorial magistrate or judge, sitting with or without a jury. A Crown Attorney presents the case on behalf of the state representing the public interest. Other interested parties may seek standing (legal status) to intervene (participate), but there is no absolute right for any individual or group to be given status. Where status is granted by the presiding coroner or magistrate, the extent of participation may be limited in scope and substance, depending on the relevance of the interest or interests to be represented.

An inquiry, usually called a public inquiry, is similar to an inquest but applies to matters concerning the good government of a province or territory or of the country.

Legislation exists to authorize the Lieutenant-Governor-in-Council to appoint a commissioner or commissioners to conduct the inquiry in the public interest.

Inquiries and inquests are public interest proceedings intended to examine the circumstances of suspicious or sudden deaths and to make recommendations to promote public safety. They are not intended to affix blame, and there are strict legal procedures in place where a presiding judge or coroner feels compelled to make statements of or respecting liability. Recommendations from an inquest or inquiry are not binding or enforceable on institutions or professionals, but they may affect public policy and clinical practice as a persuasive position. Moreover, although there are generally legislative protections in the enabling legislation and enshrined in law, the findings of an inquest or inquiry may influence subsequent or ongoing civil or criminal proceedings.

In order to minimize legal risk with respect to coroner's proceedings, the paramedic needs to be aware of and to adhere strictly to his or her reporting obligations, if any. For instance, in most jurisdictions, a paramedic will be required to report a sudden death if he or she is first on the scene. In Ontario, new legislation is in place requiring healthcare practitioners in hospitals to report gunshot wounds, although currently this does not exist in other jurisdictions.

The paramedic also needs to be aware of the jurisdictional requirements, and of the employer's policies and expectations, with respect to the need to preserve or maintain evidence at the scene. Typically, these include guidelines or requirements with respect to the state of the deceased if he or she dies at the scene or while in the care of the paramedic during treatment, during transport, or following resuscitation efforts.

In addition to evidence preservation, where reasonably possible, the paramedic needs to ensure a timely, accurate, and complete documented record of observations, treatment initiatives, including drug dosages, route of administration, frequency, and patient response, and orders from the base hospital physician, if applicable. Because death may occur after transfer of care at the receiving hospital and may not be a recognized risk on transport, the paramedic should also always ensure complete and accurate notes of circumstances of the transfer of care, including to whom, and the state of the patient upon transfer of care.

## Civil Suits and Civil Liability

Civil suits against paramedics, physicians, or allied healthcare professionals are generally framed as actions alleging malpractice or negligence. While the United States is generally viewed as a more litigious society than Canada in this regard, increasing media and public awareness of public expectations for medical and paramedic practice and treatment can reasonably result in an increased trend toward litigation in Canada.

While that expectation does not impose a standard of perfection on paramedic practice, it may mean that careless lapses in judgment resulting in breach of regulations and the applicable standards of practice may result in legal penalties. These can range from disciplinary penalties such as suspension or termination of employment, suspension or loss of certification to practice, fines, or even imprisonment if the conduct in issue is sufficiently serious that it constitutes criminal negligence. An example might be dangerous operation of an ambulance causing a motor vehicle collision resulting in death to a patient or bystander. In most cases of proven negligence, there is an expectation of compensation for damages or harm to the patient and, potentially, to the patient's family, as a result of the act or omission alleged to be the basis for the claim.

Of all of these risks, typically the one of greatest awareness and concern to paramedics is the threat of a civil suit alleging negligence, with the associated risk of a finding of negligence. It is generally understood and recognized that such a finding can be financially and professionally devastating for the professional. It can result in a damages or compensation award, the size of which will depend on the circumstances, including the nature and extent of the conduct in issue and the nature and extent of the harm, having regard to all of the circumstances surrounding the matter.

Despite this fear, and despite the numbers of law suits that may be filed, relatively few proceed to trial in Canada. Very few paramedics ever appear in a courtroom. In fact, of the law suits that are initiated, the vast majority are subsequently withdrawn, abandoned, or settled prior to trial. Despite this, the paramedic must be aware of his or her rights and responsibilities in the event he or she is named or involved in litigation alleging negligence.

## THE TORT OF NEGLIGENCE

A tort is a legal wrong resulting from an act or omission, including malpractice or negligence. This must exist to support a claim for civil liability. Second, there must be a legal recognition that a particular act or omission resulted in harm that can be compensated. This is referred to as a cause of action. Negligence by a paramedic' action(s)/omission(s) that results in patient harm will generally support a cause of action in negligence unless the act or omission or the type of harm resulting lies beyond the scope of tort law. This is rare.

Negligence by a paramedic may be generally defined as the failure to exercise the care that a reasonable and prudent paramedic in similar circumstances would have taken. In other words, if the paramedic's actions did not meet the accepted standards of practice, he or she may be found negligent in the care provided to the patient.

Four elements must exist in law to support a cause of action for negligence. First, there must be a special relationship between the parties that gives rise to a legally recognized duty of care. Second, there must be a breach of that duty. Third, the breach must result in harm or damage to the patient, and, fourth, there must be a direct and reasonably foreseeable causal connection between the conduct of the paramedic and the resulting harm to the patient.

## DUTY OF CARE (DUTY TO ACT)

As a general rule, the nature of the caregiver–patient relationship is sufficient to establish the requisite relationship to support a claim of negligence. For a paramedic, the professional relationship typically gives rise to a duty of care that is measured on both an objective standard and on a subjective standard. Objectively, the test inquires into "what a reasonable paramedic would do...". Subjectively, the test goes on to consider "...the same or similar circumstances." This two-part test allows common law to take into account any mitigating circumstances. Typically, the focus of the inquiry centres on one or more of the following in ascertaining the applicable expected standards of practice:

▪ whether the paramedic's practice conforms to existing written practice standards and guidelines;
▪ whether the paramedic's practice is consistent with the employer's written policies and procedures;
▪ the site, geographical location, type of incident, and available supports or resources, since jurisdictions may vary by resources, response, and transport times to an appropriate facility, communications access to a base hospital physician, and other factors that may affect practice capability;
▪ current industry standards, trends and developments as they may apply in a particular time frame, recognizing that a civil suit may take several years to reach court but that the applicable information is that of the time frame and the practice setting is that in existence at the time of the alleged negligent act; and
▪ type, extent, and appropriateness of training standards, recognizing that paramedics may have different levels of experience and training, including specialization or a lack thereof.

The moment a paramedic makes contact with a patient, a "duty of care" or "duty to act" has been established. This applies even if a paramedic simply asks someone at a minor motor vehicle collision if he is hurt and conducts no further assessment. In other words, it does not take much evidence to persuade the court that a paramedic–patient relationship has been established. Like the relationship between a physician and a patient, the relationship between a paramedic and a patient is one of dependence and reliance. The patient expects a high level of care and expertise and relies on the paramedics' knowledge, skills, and judgment. The paramedic has the medical knowledge to guide and direct, while the patient lacks the knowledge, with some exceptions, to disagree. This makes the patient vulnerable and places the burden of responsibility on the paramedic to provide the best care and advice possible within his or her scope of practice.

In all provinces but Quebec, there is no duty to act if the paramedic is off duty. Notwithstanding any moral or ethical sense of duty that might compel an off-duty paramedic to stop and assist, there is no legal obligation to stop, no matter how serious the incident or the injuries.

Quebec is the only province in Canada that requires that a person stop and assist. In part 1, section 2 of *The Quebec Charter of Human Rights and Freedoms*, "Every human being whose life is in peril has a right to assistance." Every person must come to the aid of anyone whose life is in peril either personally or calling for aid, by giving him the necessary and immediate physical assistance... unless it involves danger to himself or a third person, or he has another valid reason.[1]

In any event, once an off-duty paramedic stops, a duty of care is established, and she or he is now obligated to stay and provide care to the best of his or her abilities until help arrives, recognizing the off-duty paramedic does not have access to the same equipment and medical directives and cannot perform controlled acts without proper medical authority. With this commitment comes the responsibility to provide competent care and the risk of negligent liability in the event of a worsened outcome resulting from substandard care or conduct, subject to any Good Samaritan legislation that may exist in the jurisdiction. This subject will be discussed further under "Good Samaritan Laws."

## BREACH OF THE DUTY OF CARE

As discussed, the paramedic's role is primarily to respond to patients in distress. Once patient contact has been made, a duty of care or duty to act has been established. This does not mean the paramedic will provide actual care to all patients or that all patients encountered in the field will be transported to the hospital. It means that the paramedic has a responsibility to make an assessment and decisions about what, if anything, needs to be done. This may range from providing first aid and releasing the patient to extensive medical interventions followed by transport. How the paramedic performs an assessment, makes decisions, and renders care, all fall under the category of standards within that profession. The good news is that "*a standard of care and competence required, if a [paramedic] is to escape liability, is not some exalted standard presumptuously imposed by the judges, but is ordinarily the standard prevailing within the profession itself.*"[2] It is what a paramedic's peers would have done under similar circumstances. This is the premise under which "duty" is determined. To deviate from the applicable standard is a breach of duty.

Physicians are bound by several other related "duties" that have relevance to paramedic practice. For example, there is a *duty to keep full and accurate records* and a *duty to communicate with other involved professionals.*[2] In the courts, the same would be expected of paramedics. Patient care reports must be completed honestly and accurately, and as a transfer of care occurs between one paramedic and another or between the paramedic and the receiving hospital nursing or physician staff, paramedics are expected to communicate all relevant patient information as these staff members would constitute "*involved professionals*" in the continuity of care. Likewise, when a paramedic crew is called to transfer a patient from one hospital to another, they then become the newly involved professionals, and the sending hospital staff is obliged to communicate all relevant medical information.

## DAMAGE OR HARM TO THE PATIENT

Where it is established that a duty of care exists between a paramedic and a patient, and a breach of that duty occurred, the next essential element to a successful claim for civil liability is harm or damage to the patient, caused directly by the paramedic's act or omission.

However, there are other limitations or considerations applicable to a finding of civil liability. First, if the harm that resulted from the paramedic's conduct was not a reasonably foreseeable consequence of the conduct, it cannot support a finding of liability for that harm.

Second, there must be a direct causal connection between the damage or harm and the conduct of the paramedic. For instance, if it is determined that a deceased patient would have died no matter what treatment was rendered, the death cannot support a finding of civil liability against the paramedic despite deficiencies in the paramedic's treatment of the patient. However, if established practice is to splint a fractured limb distally and proximally to maintain bone alignment, a failure to do so resulting in the fracture becoming open when it was closed will result in a finding of liability on the part of the paramedic.

Third, a paramedic will not be found civilly liable for damages where the harm caused is not the damage that could reasonably be foreseen from the conduct. For instance, a paramedic may be negligent by giving a wrong medication to a patient at a scene. Because of the medication, the patient is sedated on arrival at the hospital. Another healthcare worker leaves a side rail down and the patient falls from the stretcher, sustaining injury. Despite the medication error, the paramedic may not be responsible where the second negligent act is not reasonably foreseeable. However, if the drug given in error has known side effects but, in this instance, results in a different but more severe or permanent side effect, the paramedic will likely be found negligent as the harm stems directly from the error. For example, if a paramedic inadvertently administers intravenous epinephrine instead of morphine for an elderly patient with a hip fracture and the patient subsequently dies of a cardiac dysrhythmia in the hospital, the paramedic will be held liable.

## DEFENCES TO A CLAIM OF CIVIL LIABILITY FOR NEGLIGENCE

From a legal perspective, the individual initiating the law suit (the plaintiff) bears the legal burden of proving, on a balance of probabilities, that negligence by the paramedic has occurred and has done harm. The best defence is to prove there was no breach of the duty of care. The case will turn not only on the evidence of witnesses but also on documentary evidence that supports or refutes adherence to the applicable standard. Paramedics can best protect themselves against a successful claim of negligence by

- practising in accordance with accepted standards of practice and guidelines;
- knowing and applying employer policies and procedures consistently;
- maintaining currency on practice trends and developments;
- obtaining appropriate training having regard to the geographical setting and the availability or accessibility of supporting services and resources; and
- ensuring timely, accurate, and complete documentation of all relevant observations and findings.

Realistically, a defence to an allegation of negligence generally requires that the paramedic establish that one or more of the elements of a successful claim are absent, that is, there was no duty of care, no breach of that duty, or no harm to the plaintiff, or the paramedic's practice is not the direct or proximate cause of the harm to the plaintiff. This can be accomplished by establishing, usually through witnesses or documentation of the circumstances, including expert witnesses measuring the documented or demonstrated practice of the defendant paramedic against the applicable standards of practice. An error in judgment may be insufficient to establish a breach of the duty of care where the error is not unreasonable in the circumstances.

There are two common defences against a claim of negligence that are common in medical and paramedic practices. The first is referred to as a voluntary assumption of risk, which arises from a situation in which a patient has given explicit consent to the act or omission giving rise to the harm, despite being aware of the risks associated with the acceptance or refusal of treatment. An example of this is the patient with a serious illness or injury who refuses medical treatment and transportation to a treatment facility. However, in order to establish a successful defence, the paramedic must establish that the patient had the capacity to know and understand the risk of refusing treatment or transport.

Legal capacity is the ability to understand and appreciate the nature and consequences of making a decision, including a decision to accept or refuse emergency or medical treatment. Children under the age of consent (which varies slightly by jurisdiction as shown in Table 3-1) are generally presumed to have no legal capacity to consent to or refuse medical or emergency treatment. However, exceptions may exist in healthcare where the minor is believed to be sufficiently mature and able to appreciate the consequences of that decision (e.g., birth control, abortion, non-life-threatening treatment).

While there is a presumption that an individual over the age of consent has that capacity, factors that influence mental competency may diminish or impair mental competency to the point that there is no mental capacity to consent. Factors that may diminish mental competence include but are not limited to: age, disease, diminished level of consciousness, and the influence of drugs or other sub-

| **Table 3–1** | Age of Consent for Medical Treatment in Canada |
|---|---|
| Prince Edward Island | A person must be at least 18 years of age or married to consent to surgery in a public hospital. |
| New Brunswick | The age of consent for medical treatment is 16 years of age. A younger person may consent if, in the opinion of the attending physician or dentist and one other physician or dentist, he or she is capable of understanding the nature and consequences of treatment, and the treatment is in the person's best interests with respect to continued health and well being. |
| Quebec | The age of consent is 14 years of age if the treatment is required because of the patient's state of health. For a child under 14 years of age parental consent must be obtained unless a judge orders otherwise or the child's life is in danger. |
| Saskatchewan | A person must be at least 18 years of age or married to consent to surgery in a public hospital. |
| British Columbia | A person who has reached the age of 16 years can consent to treatment if the healthcare provider has made a reasonable attempt to obtain consent from the person with parental authority and a written opinion is obtained from a second physician or dentist that the treatment is in the the person's best interests with respect to continued health and well being. |
| Other provinces | The remaining provinces have no legislation that establishes an age of consent to treatment. In common law, there is no age of consent. A minor can consent if he or she is capable of understanding the information about a treatment and of appreciating the risks and likely consequences of the treatment. |

Source: Etchells, E., Sharpe, G., Elliott, C., and Singer, P.A. Bioethics for clinicians: 3. Capacity. *Can Med Assn J.* 155(6): 657–661. Copyright © 1996 by Canadian Medical Association. Available at *http://www.cmaj.ca/misc/bio_capacity_tab1.shtml*. Accessed June 26, 2006

stances. In addition, a language or physical/communication disability barrier such as deafness can impair an individual's ability to make an informed decision in the absence of evidence that the barrier was addressed in a manner that surmounted that barrier. In certain circumstances, that barrier may require assistance of others in interpretation, or the paramedic may need to contact his or her immediate supervisor for assistance.

While a language or communication barrier can be overcome, in the absence of mental capacity or mental competence, valid consent cannot be achieved. Where competence or capacity is compromised, mental health or other substitute decision-maker legislation sets guidelines for determining capacity and for obtaining consent in instances of incapacity.

The best evidence to support that finding is for the paramedic to obtain the patient's signed release to refuse treatment, in circumstances that support a finding that the patient made an informed decision. On every call, the paramedic will be required to do some sort of capacity evaluation. The initial assessment usually includes a record of observations of the patient's ability to communicate and verbalize his or her situation, including orientation to person, place, and time, a complete assessment including vital signs, medical history, medication, and the circumstances giving rise to the call for assistance. Confusion or vagueness may resolve at the scene but should be thoroughly investigated and documented.

Supporting evidence is required for this defence. The best supporting evidence for the signed release is timely, complete, and accurate documentation of the circumstances, including of the patient's mental and physical state supporting a capacity to make the decision. Documentation should include noting the presence of any influences, witnesses, or other mitigating circumstances, including the presence or absence of language barriers and any information or instructions given to the patient or to an available responsible person present at the scene.

Implied or verbal decision making in refusing treatment or transport can be difficult or impossible to establish, although there may be factual circumstances to reasonably support such a finding in the presence of supporting witnesses. In the absence of supporting witnesses, where a patient refuses to sign or does not reasonably appear to understand the nature and impact of a decision to refuse treatment or transport, it may be necessary for the paramedic to contact the base hospital physician or immediate supervisor for advice, or to call police if applicable in the jurisdiction. A failure to do so may risk a future allegation of negligence and/or **abandonment** of a patient in need of treatment.

The second affirmative defence to a claim of negligence is that of contributory negligence on the part of the patient. This is a determination made by a court having regard to all of the circumstances. For instance, a patient who refuses or removes a splint or collar despite a clear warning may be found contributorily negligent in the event of subsequent harm resulting directly from the injury. (*Note*: There must be a finding of negligence before a finding of contributory negligence will be considered.)

In the United States, the existence of contributory negligence is a full defence to a claim of liability. In Canada, it is not a full defence. In Canada, it is likely only to result in a reduced award of compensation, based on the portion of blame accorded by the court to the actions of the patient versus the paramedic.

## VICARIOUS LIABILITY

Vicarious liability is a doctrine that applies in any employment relationship. By operation of this doctrine, an employer becomes responsible for the acts or omissions of its employees. If the employer carries liability insurance, it is the insurer who is ultimately responsible to defend and to pay, if ordered, a claim for damages. This is why most law suits name the employer, usually in addition to or in place of the employee.

The doctrine of vicarious liability has limitations, however. First, it does not protect an independent contractor. This may be important to a paramedic, as many physicians who act as Medical Directors are contracted to a hospital or medical facility and are not employees. Paramedics, who perform controlled acts such as drug administration, intravenous therapy, and advanced airway procedures, to name a few, do so at the behest of the Medical Director. In this sense, the paramedic acts as the "eyes, ears, and hands of the physician" in the field—a "physician surrogate" or "physician extender."[3] This makes the Medical Director liable or jointly liable for the controlled acts performed by the paramedic, but only to the extent the Medical Director's or designates (e.g., base hospital physician) advice or failure to adequately inform himself or herself of the circumstances before giving advice is in issue.

The paramedic remains responsible for the accuracy of observations and information provided to the Medical Director or designate. In most provinces and territories, Medical Directors are required to take out additional insurance to cover off medical oversight for paramedics working under their authority. In a negligence law suit, it is typical that both the Medical Director and the paramedics involved in a situation are named, as it may not be clear where the liability and responsibility of one ends and the other begins.

The downside of the doctrine of vicarious liability is that it is common for a physician's insurer to defend allegations of negligence against a Medical Director by attributing responsibility to the paramedic(s) in order to make the employer liable for the payment of damages in a law suit. This may manifest as allegations that any negligence was actually on the part of the paramedic, or that there was a joint liability of the paramedic that diminishes the portion of damages attributable to the Medical Director. To the extent the paramedic may be liable, vicarious liability operates to make the employer responsible for any damages payable on the part of the paramedic.

The Medical Director may be accountable for paramedic certification, maintenance of competence, the provision of continuing medical education, quality assurance, and online and offline medical direction. However, it is the responsibility of the paramedic to practise in accordance with established guidelines, policies, and procedures, and he or she is responsible for ensuring his or her own practice standards in accordance with such requirements.

Vicarious liability does not apply to the performance of care beyond the scope of the paramedic's professional employment. This means that negligent care rendered outside of the paramedic's practice (e.g., treatment or treatment advice to a friend or relative or stranger while off duty) is not covered by the employer's insurer and may result in making the paramedic personally liable for damages to the harmed person. As well, it will not protect a paramedic who undertakes treatment for which he or she is not trained and qualified, or where the harm results from willful, intentional, or criminal acts of the paramedic.

## GOOD SAMARITAN LAWS

Some but not all provinces and jurisdictions in Canada have enacted Good Samaritan laws to enshrine a formal recognition that acts or omissions undertaken in providing emergency assistance may give rise to limited or no potential liability for harm resultant from such care. Good Samaritan laws do not apply to protect persons employed and engaged in practice expressly for that purpose—for example, on-duty paramedics.

In British Columbia, Alberta, Newfoundland, Nova Scotia, Ontario, Prince Edward Island, and Saskatchewan, Good Samaritans are protected from liability unless gross negligence is shown.[2] Good Samaritan legislation typically provides that an individual is not legally required to act in an emergency situation (except in Quebec), but if he or she does so, he or she is relieved of liability for negligence in the course of so doing. The underlying rationale is to promote emergency intervention by heathcare providers by ensuring it will not result in a successful claim for malpractice or negligence.

A paramedic who is a member of a governing body may still, however, be responsible to his or her governing body for the care rendered. He or she remains responsible to act in accordance with the established rules of professional practice and recognized standards of practice, but having regard to all of the circumstances, such as availability of resources, specialized knowledge or skills, and so on.

It is worth noting that even in jurisdictions without Good Samaritan legislation, there are few if any successful law suits in Canada for care rendered gratuitously by individuals, including off-duty paramedics, in an emergency situation.

## THE CIVIL TORT OF ASSAULT AND BATTERY

*Black's Law Dictionary* (6th Edition, 1990) defines **assault** as the "willful attempt or threat to inflict injury upon the person of another, when coupled with an apparent present ability so to do, and any intentional display of force such as would give the victim reason to fear or expect immediate bodily harm." Battery is also a form of application of illegal force.

For paramedics, allegations of assault and battery typically arise from the commencement of treatment without consent, or unwanted touching at a scene where the patient resists or refuses treatment. However, as a general rule, emergency or life-threatening circumstances will not give rise to a finding of tort liability in the absence of a clear refusal of treatment by a patient who is mentally, physically, and legally capable in the circumstances of giving or withholding consent to treatment. In order to maintain the standards of practice, the paramedic must consider all emergency circumstances on their individual merits. If there is any doubt about the capacity or capability of a patient to refuse or resist treatment, the prudent paramedic should contact, if possible, additional emergency or social services personnel to assist in assessing and defusing or appropriately responding to the patient circumstance.

## Professional Liability

Professional liability arises only in the context of a self-regulating profession. Paramedic exposure to potential professional liability can occur only in those provinces in which the paramedic is licensed or certified to practise by a governing regulatory body, or where the paramedic may also hold credentials of a regulated healthcare professional.

Governing bodies are established and mandated to protect the public interest by setting and enforcing applicable standards of practice. As part of that legislated mandate, they are given powers to enforce and sanction professional misconduct and incompetence, including incapacity to practise.

A regulated healthcare professional is responsible for his or her own conduct and practice. Physicians and other healthcare providers such as nurses are self-regulated and therefore liable for their own practice. However, the regulated healthcare professional may also be held accountable or liable for certain acts of others arising due to substandard supervision or a failure to adequately determine the skill level, competence, or knowledge of another individual with whom he or she has a shared responsibility for treatment. This is particularly true in paramedic practice where the controlling physician must rely on the paramedic's expertise to assess and direct treatment of a patient at a scene or during transport. It also applies, where Advanced Care Paramedics (ACPs) are paired with Primary Care Paramedics (PCPs). The ACP, having a higher level of medical training than the PCP, has greater responsibility for the patient care and may have some professional responsibility for the practice of the PCP.

Most paramedics in Canada receive their medical delegation from a Medical Director or designate who delegates a course of treatment. Where the delegated course of treatment does not meet the standard, the Medical Director may be held accountable. However, the paramedic will also be held accountable if the physician gives an order that the paramedic knew or ought to have known was wrong. In a situation where the paramedic fails to carry out written or verbal orders from the physician correctly, the physician is not accountable for the acts or omissions of the paramedic and can pass the civil liability on to the paramedic.

While each practitioner is responsible for his or her own practice, the physician has an added responsibility to know and respect the capacity and capability of the paramedic. The physician must ensure he or she does not expect or assume capacity in the paramedic to perform beyond their accepted scope of practice or to fail to recognize limitations in skill, knowledge, or training relevant to the circumstances of patient care. This shared responsibility can strain the relationship between the paramedic and the physician, as it may result in a perceived mistrust of the paramedic practice by the physician, or a tendency to micro-manage a patient in an online medical control situation.

In any event, a finding of professional liability by a governing body can result in discipline, limitations on practice, or suspension or revocation of certification to practice. It is frequently imposed in addition to employment, civil or criminal liability, or any combination.

## Criminal Liability

Criminal liability is the least likely legal risk for a paramedic in the course of his or her practice. A finding of criminal negligence may result in a criminal conviction, such as dangerous driving in the event of a traffic collision in the course of an ambulance response. Assault charges can stem from a patient altercation to restrain an out-of-control individual. However, such charges and convictions arising from paramedic practice are rare in the absence of intentional or extreme conduct, as circumstances in emergency treatment will generally mitigate against such a finding.

A likelier source of criminal liability for the paramedic stems from intentional criminal acts while on duty, such as theft of drugs or theft from a patient. To avoid successful criminal allegations, the paramedic should be careful to observe applicable policies and procedures for dealing with ambulance equipment and medical supplies and with personal possessions of patients.

## PATIENT CONFIDENTIALITY, CONSENT, AND DOCUMENTATION

There are many specific practice considerations of importance to the practising paramedic. Among the most important considerations in patient relations are: patient confidentiality, patient consent to treatment, and appropriate documentation standards to reflect and record appropriate care and treatment.

## Patient Confidentiality

Paramedics in all jurisdictions of Canada are subject to a number of statutes and regulations protecting patient confidentiality and privacy of personal information, including medical, information. A paramedic who releases or discloses private patient information inappropriately will be held professionally and personally liable, whether or not there was any intention. Patient confidentiality is a professional duty and ethical responsibility, with recognized legal exceptions to facilitate treatment and care while maintaining reasonable patient expectations of confidentiality. In all jurisdictions, legislation prescribes protection of privacy and the circumstances in which personal information, including in particular health information, can be released.

As a rule, paramedics should treat all patient information as privileged, or confidential, including information such as health insurance policy numbers that do not directly identify the patient. Protection against disclosure includes information in any format, be it verbal, written, or electronic. All patient documentation, therefore, must never be left in the open. It should be reasonably secured such that it is inaccessible to persons who have no right to it without express legal access. Similarly, radio or cell phone communications are subject to considerations of patient confidentiality. It is therefore expected that paramedics refrain, where possible, from using a patient's name or identifying information in such communications.

### RELEASE OF INFORMATION

Authorization to release patient information generally requires consent from the patient, unless it falls within a legal exception. Legislation varies by jurisdiction, but generally, exceptions that may allow for the release or sharing of patient medical and personal information typically include

- sharing information with other healthcare professionals for the purpose of ensuring appropriate treatment and continuity of care;
- where required by law (including mandatory reporting situations such as suspected child abuse), or as part of an investigation into ambulance service delivery or paramedic practice by the designated provincial or territorial authority responsible for oversight of Ambulance services;
- where required to advance or in the course of a legal proceeding brought about by legal process (e.g., subpoena , warrant, or court order), or to aid in an investigation by a law enforcement agency that is likely to result in a legal proceeding; and
- in emergency or other circumstances where the health or safety of the patient or others is at risk (e.g., a patient states she is going to kill herself and wants to kill others).

Because all patient information a paramedic obtains as a result of his or her duties is confidential, the paramedic must satisfy himself or herself that release or disclosure in any circumstance is in accordance with legal exceptions and conforms, where applicable, to employer guidelines, policies, and procedures. When in doubt, it is expected the paramedic will consult a supervisor for direction.

### PRIVACY-RELATED LEGISLATION

Healthcare professionals, including paramedics, are required to maintain acceptable standards of protecting patient confidentiality and privacy, governed generally by professional ethical guidelines and standards of practice. However, there is applicable and stringent federal and provincial legislation in all jurisdictions. In particular, there are specific rules and requirements with respect to the use of and access to healthcare information of an individual. Examples of specific legislation in differing jurisdictions include the following:

- Federal: *The Personal Information Protection and Electronic Documents Act (PIPEDA)*
- Federal: *The Privacy Act*
- Federal: *The Access to Information Act*
- British Columbia: *Freedom of Information and Protection of Privacy Act; Security and Privacy Guidelines for Health Information Systems* (COACH 1995)
- Alberta: *Health Information Act*
- Saskatchewan: *Health Information Protection Act*
- Manitoba: *Personal Health Information Act*
- Ontario: *Personal Health Information Protection Act (P-HIPA)*
- Quebec: *An Act Respecting the Protection of Personal Information in the Private Sector; An Act Respecting Access to Documents Held by Public Bodies and the Protection of Personal Information*

In addition to meeting legal requirements for use and disclosure of personal and healthcare information of an individual, the paramedic needs to respect the sensitivity of such information. Accordingly, it is recommended that legal disclosure be handled carefully, as certain negative phrases or statements may be perceived as insulting or disrespectful, even to the extent of defamatory or discriminatory, dependent on situational facts and circumstances.

## Consent

As discussed previously in this chapter, all medical care and treatment requires patient consent. All individuals in Canada have rights enshrined in common law, and in statutes such as the *Canadian Charter of Rights and Freedoms*, which states:

> Everyone has the right to life, liberty and security of the person and the right not to be deprived thereof except in accordance with the principles of fundamental justice.[4]

Based on common law and statute, therefore, the law recognizes that medical intervention or the performance of an invasive procedure on a person without his or her consent, even in emergency circumstances, may be a violation of a patient's fundamental rights.

Provincial acts, such as the Ontario Health Care Consent Act, give greater specificity to the nature and requirements of healthcare consent. It is therefore essential that the paramedic understand the importance of consent and its impact on all treatment-related decisions. For clarity, all patient treatment requires patient consent or the consent of an individual empowered by law to give consent for or in place of the patient, except in special circumstances that impose a legal ability or obligation to treat. Treatment in the absence of consent, substitute consent or legal justification can result in legal liability for breach of patient rights.

## INFORMED CONSENT

A patient has the right to be informed as to the nature of care or treatment to be provided, why it is required, and whether or not there are any risks to receiving or refusing the treatment. Consent may be express or implicit. **Express consent** may be verbal or written. **Implied consent** is typically demonstrated by acquiescence or a failure to object.

Where a patient is conscious and capable, a paramedic is required to seek consent to treatment, even if it is simply a verbal "yes," or nonverbal such as nodding of the head in the affirmative or acquiescing to and cooperating with treatment without complaint. However, in order for consent to be legally valid, it must also be *informed*.

**Informed consent** requires that a patient be given sufficient information about the need for and particulars of the planned care or treatment to understand the consequences of accepting or refusing it. It further requires that the patient have the capacity and competence to understand the information and to make a decision to accept or decline care or treatment. Patients whose mental competence is compromised by disease (including mental illness), age, diminished level of consciousness, or drugs or other substances have no legal capacity to consent to or refuse treatment.

In terms of practice implications for the paramedic, this means some patients are unable to give a valid or informed consent to accept or decline treatment. Such circumstances include but are not limited to
- minors (below the age of healthcare consent applicable in that jurisdiction),
- diabetics who are hypoglycemic or hyperglycemic,
- individuals who are confused,
- patients with a Glasgow Coma Scale (GCS) score of less than 15,
- individuals who are intoxicated or under the influence of a toxic substance (usually drugs or alcohol),
- persons who are agitated or in shock,
- those who have an active mental illness or debility, or
- persons who are otherwise unable to appreciate the consequences of a treatment decision.

Also, as discussed previously in this chapter, individuals who have a language or communication barrier, while they may be competent and capable, may not be able to give a valid consent unless the barrier has been appropriately addressed through interpretation or other means that allows the individual to understand the information.

Where a patient is unconscious, or mentally incompetent and apparently in need of life saving interventions or care, the paramedic can rely on a legal presumption of implied and valid consent. This presumption assumes the patient would, if capable, consent to the intervention in circumstances that would otherwise result in death or serious harm with a risk of death if left untreated.

This presumption is generally applicable when three criteria are met:
1. the person is incapable of understanding the treatment by way of incompetence or altered level of awareness,
2. the person is at risk, and if the treatment is not administered, the person could suffer serious bodily harm or death, and
3. it is not possible to obtain a consent or refusal on the person's behalf from a substitute decision-maker (like a relative), or the delay required to do so would put the person at risk of serious bodily harm or death.

An example of such circumstance applies with respect to a diabetic patient with a depressed level of consciousness and confirmed hypoglycemia. He or she may be awake and agitated but not competent to make decisions about his or her care, and a failure to treat will result in death.

Implied consent is not appropriate for elective procedures or for care or treatment that may be recommended but not required. As well, if the patient recovers legal capacity to make or withdraw informed consent (e.g., the hypoglycemic after initial treatment), the presumption of implied consent no longer applies and consent can be withdrawn.

## INVOLUNTARY CONSENT

In the absence of informed or implied consent, a paramedic can seek **involuntary consent** if necessary for the safety and security of the patient or others. The most common example of this is the exercise of police powers to place an individual in custody to require the patient to be forcibly transported to an appropriate medical facility for medical attention. This usually, but not always, occurs as a result of suspected psychiatric incapacity. All provinces and territories have legislation that provides for involuntary committal for psychiatric observation in particular circumstances. An example is taken from section 10 of the New Brunswick Mental Health Act:

> The patient has threatened or attempted, or is threatening or attempting, to cause harm to himself or herself, has behaved or is behaving in a way that causes or is likely to cause another person harm or is causing another person to fear harm from the person, or has shown or is showing a lack of competence to care for himself or herself.

Paramedics must be familiar with the guidelines, acts, and regulations applicable in their practice jurisdiction.

## SUBSTITUTE DECISION-MAKERS

*Minors.*  As stated previously, a minor under the age of consent, which varies by jurisdiction between 16 and 18, are generally presumed to have no legal capacity to consent to medical care and treatment. However, in some circumstances minors at age 16 (or younger in some jurisdictions and in some circumstances) can legally consent to accept or decline medical treatment if a parent is not available at the time, and if they can demonstrate a full and competent appreciation of the risks associated with their decision. (If in doubt as to capacity, the paramedic should assume a minor under the age of 16 cannot consent.) A parent or legal guardian is required to give consent on behalf of the minor. However, a paramedic can transport a minor in the absence of a parent or legal guardian where the paramedic believes emergency care or transport is required.

*Mentally Incompetent Adults.* Providing care to a patient who has a cognitive disability; is otherwise impaired by virtue of disease, injury, extreme anxiety, or mental illness; or is under the influence of a toxic substance can be challenging to a paramedic. The paramedic cannot assume the patient is capable or incapable of making decisions but must carefully assess the patient through interview and observation.

If the paramedic reaches the conclusion that the patient is not capable of making informed decisions, he or she should first attempt to get consent from a legal substitute decision-maker (depending on circumstances, this may be a spouse, child, parent, or legal guardian), or, if necessary, the police. Several jurisdictions in Canada have legislation that determines who can act as a substitute decision-maker and in what circumstances.

As a last resort, the paramedic may forcibly treat or transport an incompetent adult, but only in a life-threatening situation.

## PRISONERS AND PATIENTS-IN-CUSTODY

A patient in a psychiatric or correctional facility has the same rights as others with respect to treatment and care decisions. The same tests and exceptions apply. For example, a patient under arrest, having recently been subdued by a Taser™, may still have the needle probes in his skin. If trained and authorized to do so, a paramedic may be asked to help remove these probes prior to moving the individual. However, if the patient refuses and demands transport to hospital, the fact he is in custody does not supercede his right to make that decision.

## REFUSAL OF CARE OR TRANSPORT

Also, as previously discussed in this chapter, a mentally competent adult has the legal right to refuse care or transport, or both. This is true even where the refusal could result in consequences up to and including death, but that does not relieve the paramedic of all responsibility. In fact, refusals of service have a high potential to lead to allegations of wrongdoing by the paramedic, with potential resultant legal liability ranging from employment consequences to criminal charges.

Like consent, a refusal of care or treatment must be informed and legally valid. Most systems require that the patient or, if the patient is a minor or lacks capacity, a com-

petent substitute decision-maker, sign a refusal of service form. For the protection of the paramedic, however, refusals of service require as much, and arguably better, documentation than a call that results in transport. The mnemonic C-I-A can be useful in assisting the paramedic to determine the appropriate course of action when a patient refuses care or transport against the advice of the paramedic. The system developed by the Regional Base Hospital Program for Southeastern Ontario has become a widely accepted recommended practice, in addition to the charting aspects identified by the province's Ministry of Health as minimum requirements for a refusal of service.

C stands for capacity. The paramedic must first determine whether the patient has the capacity, including the communication and language facility, to understand the circumstances and to make an informed decision. A patient signature on a refusal of service form is not valid evidence to support a decision to decline transport if the patient lacks basic command of the language, unless other compelling evidence exists to support a reasonable conclusion that the patient understood. For example, receiving a coherent reply to the question "Do you know what could happen to you if I leave here without treating you or taking you to the hospital?" provides evidence that the patient understands the language, can answer coherently, and has a rational appreciation of why you may be concerned.

I stands for informed. The patient must be explicitly warned of the reasonably foreseeable worst-case consequence of a refusal of service. It is not sufficient to document that a patient was advised of the risks. It is necessary to specify what risks were mentioned. For instance, the worst-case reasonably foreseeable consequences of a decision to refuse treatment for a finger injury may include pain, deformity, and permanent loss of function. In contrast, a patient who is treated for but rapidly recovers from acute hypoglycemia and refuses transport, may risk a life-threatening relapse. In such cases, Medical Directives may provide further steps for the paramedic to take to ensure that the likelihood of a relapse is minimized and that the patient and/or caregiver knows he or she should call again for assistance should a relapse occur.

A stands for action. The paramedic should try to determine what the patient may do once the paramedics have left. In most cases, patients say they will see their family doctor, or will call 911 if further problems should arise, or that a friend or relative will assist them. The paramedic should ask if that friend or relative will be remaining with the patient and should fully document all answers given by the patient.

A signature without supporting documentation is not sufficient to alleviate a paramedic's potential liability in the event there is subsequent injury or harm as a result of the refusal of medical care and treatment. Combined, if all elements of C-I-A are addressed and fully documented, even in point form, it is reasonably established that informed refusal of service took place.

## OTHER LEGAL COMPLICATIONS RELATED TO CONSENT

A failure to obtain a legally valid and informed consent from a patient can result in allegations of civil liability for negligence, as previously discussed, and/or to a law suit and criminal liability arising from allegations of abandonment, **forcible confinement**, and assault. However, criminal charges in these circumstances are rare and likely to be pursued only in exceptional circumstances supporting the conclusion that the paramedic acted willfully or purposefully in violating the rights and wishes of the patient.

*Abandonment.*  Section 215 of the Criminal Code states that everyone has a legal duty to provide necessities of life to a person under his or her care if that person is unable, by reason of illness, mental disorder, or other cause, to safely care for himself or herself without the care and supervision being provided, or is otherwise unable to provide himself or herself with the necessities of life.

Once a paramedic makes direct contact on site with a patient, there is a relationship from which a duty of care arises. Improperly terminating care that has been started, or turning over a patient to an inappropriate or unqualified care provider who does not have the capacity or means to continue that care can constitute patient abandonment giving rise to serious civil and/or criminal consequences. For these reasons, there are a variety of provincial and territorial protocols and regulations that are existent to address EMS transfer of care. For example, a paramedic could be found liable for abandonment for leaving a patient with Alzheimer's disease on an ambulance stretcher in a hospital corridor without ensuring proper delegation to the care and supervision of a responsible person, if the stretcher tipped over or the patient climbed down or fell off. Another example would be that of a paramedic who elects to intubate a patient, then hands the patient off to a volunteer firefighter without an appropriate level of medical training.

*Assault.*  Section 265 of the Criminal Code makes it an offence if, without the consent of another person, the paramedic applies force intentionally to that other person, directly or indirectly, or even if the paramedic attempts or threatens, by an act or a gesture, to apply force to another person, if that action gives the other person reasonable grounds to believe that the threat will be carried out.

Obviously, striking a patient without legal justification would be viewed as criminal assault. However, allegations of assault by a paramedic most frequently arise from situations in which the paramedic inappropriately and forcibly restrains or threatens to restrain a patient in order to initiate treatment. Use of reasonable force in life-threatening circumstances where a patient does not have the competence or capacity to consent or to refuse is not assault. For instance, a patient with a severe life-threatening head injury resulting in incapacity, aggression, and confusion may appropriately require restraint in order to initiate treatment and transport.

*Forcible Confinement.*  Section 279 of the Criminal Code makes it an offence for anyone to unlawfully confine, imprison, or forcibly seize (take) a person against his or her will, including forcible transport to a hospital or medical facility despite an express and informed refusal of care. An adult patient who is conscious, alert, and oriented and answers all questions coherently and with an appreciation for risks can refuse care. If, despite determining that a patient is competent, the paramedic forces the patient into the ambulance for transport to the hospital, the paramedic could be charged with making forcible confinement.

There is no forcible confinement in circumstances where a paramedic forcibly transports a patient who lacks the legal capacity to make an informed decision to refuse care. For example, a patient under the influence of alcohol or drugs and showing signs of decreased level of consciousness may lack capacity to refuse treatment. The paramedic should seek the assistance of law enforcement personnel to assist but may transport forcibly if assistance is not readily available and treatment is necessary to preserve life. In this scenario, the paramedic should be diligent to ensure—thorough documentation of the circumstances, including the patient condition and responses—the reasons for transport and treatment, and that all steps are taken to attempt to gain compliance prior to forcibly transporting and treating. These decisions are not to be made lightly, having regard to the right of a competent and legally capable patient to refuse care and/or transport, even in life-threatening circumstances.

## USE OF FORCE AND PATIENT RESTRAINT

There are circumstances that legally justify a paramedic to use force in self-defence or, in very specific circumstances, to provide care essential for the preservation of life. In either case, the paramedic should only do so if all other recourses have failed and if police presence is not available.

The capability to use some force in necessary and life-threatening circumstances to facilitate treatment is articulated in some provincial legislation. For example, Section 7 of Ontario Health Care Consent Act indicates that there is a duty of a caregiver to restrain or confine a person when immediate action is necessary to prevent serious bodily harm to the person or to others. The type of force used can be physical or chemical, including the use of sedation.

# Documentation

Documentation is an important part of paramedic practice. The quality of the record has extensive implications for the patient and for the paramedic. The record may be reviewed by colleagues and medical personnel to make treatment decisions, by the employer and/or the Medical Director in maintaining standards of quality assurance, by administrators, by patients, by coroners investigating patient mortality, and by lawyers preparing to pursue or defend a legal proceeding. It is necessary for communication, continuity of care, professional accountability, auditing of practice standards and protocols, and for clinical or evaluative research.

Patient care, or ambulance call, reports are developed to serve many functions. The mnemonic CLeAR can be of help in remembering these purposes, and it can also remind the paramedic of one of the most important requirements on any documentation: It must be clear and legible. CLeAR stands for Clinical, Legal, Administrative, and Research.

**Clinical**: Paramedic documentation forms a part of the patient's hospital record and is integral to initiating treatment and to the continuity of care. Information such as chief complaint, past and present medical history, medication allergies, systems-based assessment findings of both objective and subjective nature, procedures or interventions performed, and drugs given have obvious importance. The clinical documentation is also used for quality assurance purposes to ascertain paramedic skills inventory and ensure compliance with protocols and accepted standards.

**Legal:** Patient care documentation also forms part of the legal record. It may be used in evidence supporting or defending claims against medical (including the paramedic's) practice. It may provide documentary evidence at inquests or inquiries, in criminal or civil trials, or in professional proceedings, including paramedic certification reviews focused on quality of patient care and compliance with established standards of practice.

**Administrative**: The administrative information includes demographic data such as the patient's name, age, address, and location of the call. It also includes mileage, all response times, service information, and more. This information can be used for billing purposes, to assist with planning for future EMS development (such as where to locate new ambulance stations or to develop vehicle deployment strategies), or to elucidate the need for revisions of employer policies and procedures.

**Research:** Virtually all data on a report, including demographic and clinical documentation, can be very useful for research purposes. They can be used for both retrospective and prospective research to determine the efficacy of paramedic interventions, test new treatments, and help shape the future of paramedic practice and EMS systems.

The primary importance of documentation for the practising paramedic is in terms of clinical practice and for legal purposes. In meeting the objectives of effective clinical, legal, administrative, and research use, patient charting must meet, as a minimum, the following standards:

- It must be accurate, true, clear, concise, complete and legible.
- Forms must be completed as soon after a call as practical. If there are any delays in completing the documentation, it should be noted on the report when it was actually completed.
- If the document is written (as opposed to electronic), blue or black ink should be used, depending on local policy, and enough pressure applied to reach through

multiple copies if it is a carbon-based or pressure-sensitive multiple copy document.
- Entries should be recorded in chronological order utilizing a 24-hour clock system, unless policies specifically dictate otherwise.
- The document should be distributed to the appropriate locations as soon as possible, with appropriate measures taken to maintain the security and confidentiality of the information.
- Errors or changes should be clearly marked in a manner consistent with applicable policy or industry standards. For instance, it is common practice to draw a single line through a documentation error and initial the change. Whiteout or other erasure methods must not be used, as any indicators of tampering will reduce the credibility of the document and of the recorder.

Documentation should be stored in a secure manner, whether paper based or electronic, such that it is not accessible except to those with the legal right to its access. In either case, there are legislative requirements and employer policies that stipulate how long the record must be kept (commonly five years or more). After the applicable record retention period has expired, ongoing confidentiality processes typically require that documentation be destroyed.

# OTHER PRACTICE CONSIDERATIONS

## Certification to Practise

Each province or territory in Canada has requirements for some form of certification to practise for paramedics and to regulate paramedic practice. This varies by jurisdiction, ranging from proof of having met prescribed educational requirements, to elaborate systems of annual recertification and continuing medical education requirements. Each government regulates under what conditions an otherwise qualified paramedic is permitted to practise.

Typically, certification can take one of two forms: It can be akin to registration—a one- time credentialling that certifies the paramedic has met prescribed testing to qualify him or her for employment. Alternatively, certification can be akin to certification or licensure after employment has begun, but prior to permission to perform patient care activities. The second is more common in Canada and is the one more commonly referred to as certification status.

Certification is conferred on an individual by a delegated authority under provincial or territorial control. For example, Ontario paramedics must certify on an annual basis with a local or Regional Base Hospital designated by the province's Emergency Health Service Branch. In Alberta, licensure is controlled by the Alberta College of Paramedics, with an established structure providing for self-regulation. In New Brunswick, paramedics must maintain registration with the Paramedic Association of New Brunswick (PANB).

Various means of controlling the right to practise as a paramedic exist, ranging from direct government licensing, to self-regulating professional colleges, to professional associations. This may occur in two distinct forms of certification: a pre-employment registration and validation of credentials process, or an ongoing maintenance of clinical competency certification process.

## Scope of Practice

Scope of practice refers to the range of knowledge, skills, and abilities that is expected of a competently trained paramedic for a level of practice within a given province or territory in Canada. The scope of practice may infer a general consensus (or position statement) on expected scope of practice and includes applicable legislation or regulations that detail what is actually permitted in the specific jurisdiction.

The National Occupational Competency Profile for Paramedics (referred to in Chapter 1), for example, is a document that was created to reach consensus on the competencies expected for each of the three levels of paramedic practice in Canada today. The three levels are Primary, Advanced, and Critical Care Paramedic. This profile does not have the force of being a standard or a regulation, since it is the responsibility of each jurisdiction to determine how to regulate the actual scope of practice. However, in reaching consensus on what should or ought to be the scope of practice for each level, interjurisdictional labour mobility for paramedics becomes possible, since there is at least a common language used in defining this ideal scope of practice.

With respect to legislated practice considerations, it remains the responsibility of each province or territory (or in the case of the military, by the Canadian Forces Health Services) to define in statute and regulation the scope of practice and how it will be regulated and enforced. For example, the title of Emergency Medical Technician– Paramedic, in Alberta, is regulated by the Alberta College of Paramedics, which, in turn, has its authority under provincial legislation (The Alberta Health Professions Act).

## Medical Direction and Practice of Delegated or Controlled Medical Acts

Medical Direction, also referred to as Medical Oversight, is an essential component of quality EMS care. The Medical Director delegates controlled acts through online or offline control. With respect to Basic Life Support (BLS) skills, the paramedic is not required to seek online medical control or permission to proceed.

The geography of Canada has somewhat shaped a low historical reliance on online medical direction. Vast geographical areas continue to have unreliable or nonexistent cell-phone and radio communications. In such areas, the ability to access direct contact with a physician is severely limited. For this reason, some medical directives that normally require the paramedic to contact a base hospital physician for a direct order may contain a caveat allowing the paramedic to perform the controlled act if all attempts to communicate with the physician have failed.

## Mandatory Reporting Requirements

Paramedics are subject to a number of mandatory reporting requirements to external agencies. These requirements are determined and regulated at the provincial or territorial level. For example, every province and territory requires paramedics to report suspected cases of child maltreatment and neglect, although the exact requirements vary by jurisdiction. Paramedics must know their reporting obligations as established in their respective jurisdiction. Specific details can be found in the following legislation:

- British Columbia Child, Family and Community Service Act
- Alberta Child, Youth and Family Enhancement Act and Child Welfare Act
- Saskatchewan Child and Family Services Act
- Manitoba Child and Family Services Act
- Ontario Child and Family Services Act
- Quebec Youth Protection Act
- New Brunswick Family Services Act
- Nova Scotia Children and Family Services Act
- Prince Edward Island Child Protection Act
- Newfoundland and Labrador
- Yukon Territory Child and Family Services Act
- Northwest Territories Child and Family Services Act
- Nunavut Territory Children's Act

Reporting requirements for other matters, whether mandatory or not, vary by jurisdiction. For example, suspected domestic violence is not something that paramedics are required to specifically report to an external agency (such as the police). However, the presence of children in a suspected domestic violence situation may require reporting as a potential situation of neglect or emotional abuse for those children.

Ontario recently enacted (effective September 1, 2005) the Mandatory Gunshot Wounds Reporting Act. Ontario hospitals and healthcare facilities are now required to report to police, as soon as is practical, the name of a patient with a gunshot wound, if known, and the location of the reporting facility. It is the first legislation in Canada that acknowledges a potential connection between gunshot wounds and serious criminal activity placing public safety at risk. In other jurisdictions, there continues to be no legal requirement to report gunshot wounds, and to do so constitutes a breach of patient confidentiality.

There are now also laws for reporting of suspected elder abuse in nursing homes and institutions in all provinces and territories. British Columbia, Saskatchewan, Quebec, New Brunswick, Prince Edward Island, and all three territories have legislation permitting voluntary reporting, but reporting is not mandatory. In these jurisdictions, there are interprovincial variations to the extent those making the allegations are protected from liability. In contrast, Alberta,

Manitoba, Ontario, Nova Scotia, and Newfoundland and Labrador have mandatory reporting legislation, although in some cases, the mandate extends only to nursing home staff, and not specifically to paramedics. Specific reporting requirements can be found in the following applicable legislation:

- British Columbia Adult Guardianship Act
- Alberta Protection for Persons in care Act
- Saskatchewan Victims of Domestic Violence Act
- Manitoba Protection for Persons in Care Act
- Ontario Nursing Homes Act
- Quebec Charte de Droits et Liberties de la Personne
- New Brunswick Family Services Act
- Nova Scotia Adult Protection Act
- Prince Edward Island Adult Protection Act
- Newfoundland and Labrador Neglected Adults Welfare Act
- Yukon Territory Adult Protection and Decision Making Act being Schedule A to the Decision-Making Support and Protection to Adults Act
- Northwest Territories Family Violence Act
- Nunavut Guardianship and Trustees Act

Other situations that may have mandatory or voluntary reporting requirements include sexual assaults, animal bites, and certain infectious diseases. The variation of reporting requirements, investigatory procedures, and enforcement mechanisms between provincial and territorial jurisdictions illustrates the complexity of the operation of the legal system in Canada. It speaks to the need for a paramedic to be aware and conversant with the various mandatory reporting laws and guidelines applicable to his or her specific practice jurisdiction. In addition, whether or not there is a specific reporting requirement in a province or territory for a given situation, there is an overriding professional expectation and obligation that the paramedic will accurately and completely document all relevant observations and findings and consult with his or her immediate supervisor for guidance.

## Notification of Infectious Disease Exposure

Some provinces, such as Ontario, have legislation to protect medical and paramedic personnel who may have been exposed to infectious diseases. Ontario's Health Protection and Promotion Act and Ontario Regulation 166/03 offer some protection rights to emergency workers, including paramedics.

Jurisdictions do not typically provide for the testing of patients for communicable diseases against their will, absent a court order in specific circumstances. However, many jurisdictions require that paramedics and other healthcare professionals be informed if they have been exposed to a patient with a confirmed diagnosis of a communicable disease. Most provinces and territories also have occupational health and safety legislation that requires the employer to designate a specific contact person or internal protocol for reporting possible exposures, so as to permit post-exposure assessment, documentation, and, where indicated, prophylaxis.

## Transport

While the term Ambulance Driver no longer accurately describes the scope of practice for Canadian paramedics, it nevertheless captures a significant aspect of the job that cannot be ignored. The operation of ambulances and the specific regulations governing how they are to be equipped and labelled rests at the provincial or territorial level. Drivers' licensing requirements for paramedics, for example, varies by province or territory. However, The Criminal Code of Canada includes some driving-related offences that are in addition to the provincial considerations. For example, impaired driving is a criminal code violation. A conviction could preclude a paramedic from working as a paramedic in Canada, unless he or she had been granted a pardon.

The driver of an emergency vehicle must operate the vehicle safely and courteously at all times. This is a legal requirement, and a public expectation, as the public looks to paramedics as role models for safety. In emergency situations of a life-threatening nature, use of audible and visual warning systems may assist paramedics with expedient travel, and all Canadian jurisdictions have provincial or territorial laws that govern motor vehicle operation and specific rules respecting emergency vehicles. These laws elaborate, for example, on whether or not certain exemptions apply to paramedics when using warning systems. Examples include legislated rights to exceed the posted speed limit; the right to travel the wrong way on posted one-way streets, to proceed cautiously through a red light, or to pass on a paved shoulder. Paramedics must be familiar with the specific exemptions and expectations as they pertain to the jurisdiction where they are working, including limitations on those exemptions (e.g., an ambulance can proceed *cautiously* through a red light, having regard to traffic and other impediments and risks). Paramedics must also adhere to service policies and procedures which may place additional restrictions on such things as speed or how to proceed at stops signs and traffic lights.

Emergency vehicle operating privileges could be abused and could result in liability to the paramedic, not to mention danger to the public. An example would be imprudent use of speed, or unreasonably using warning systems in less than emergent cases. Provincial and territorial laws generally do permit paramedics to exceed the posted speed limit in emergencies, but the Criminal Code still applies with respect to a driver's responsibilities. While speeding in a school zone en route to an emergency may not result in a provincial offence, it could result in a criminal code charge if a child is struck, as prudence should be used in weighing the laws permitting speeding against those requiring due diligence.

## CHOICE OF PATIENT DESTINATION

As an overall guiding principle, and in the absence of specific direction or requirements to the contrary, patients should be transported to the closest, most appropriate hospital. However, this is not as simple as it might sound. The decision is a complex balance between the patient's request (if he or she has one), the patient's needs, and the authority or degree of control given to dispatchers over operational criteria.

Often, a patient has a prior notion of where he or she wishes to be transported. Much like any other decision regarding health care, it is generally assumed that patients have the right to make such determinations. To the extent that this is possible, patient requests must be taken into consideration. Geographically, this may not be possible, of course, especially in the instance of small communities with only one hospital, and with the next closest hospital being unreasonably distant to consider under routine circumstances.

In assessing the appropriate destination, the paramedic must take into consideration the nature of the patient illness or injury and of the patient status. If a dialysis patient requires urgent care and there is a choice of two hospitals, both being an equal distance from the paramedic's current location, the one offering dialysis services is the obvious best choice. Specialized services such as obstetric care, neonatology care, trauma care, emergency care, stroke and cardiac intervention services, and burn care are often regionalized. In many cases, local and regional protocols are prepared to allow for bypassing closer hospitals in favour of specialized service for patients that meet protocol guidelines. Paramedics must be aware of what protocols are in place in the jurisdiction where they work.

In addition, most systems vest some degree of control over the destination decision with dispatchers. For example, as discussed in Chapter 1, a given hospital may be experiencing overcrowding and can no longer accept lower-acuity patients or may already be coping with a major incident or disaster situation unknown to the paramedic. In that situation, the paramedic will likely be directed by the dispatcher to an alternative destination. The authority to direct to an alternative destination is normally a delegated authority under a provincial regulation.

## TRANSFER OF CARE

Assuming that a patient is to be transported, the paramedic's responsibility for the patient does not end with a verbal report to the triage nurse. The transfer of care may begin at this point, and in fact, once a hospital chart has been started, however, the paramedics involved are still partially responsible for ongoing assessment and, possibly, for ongoing care. A complete transfer of care occurs only when the patient has been physically moved from the ambulance stretcher to a hospital bed and all pertinent patient infor-

mation has been relayed to the nurse or most responsible physician. Paramedics should consult with local medical directives and policies and procedures for further clarification on transfer of care issues.

## ISSUES RELATED TO FEE FOR AMBULANCE SERVICE

Although the right to health care in Canada is afforded some federal status accessible to all Canadians under the Canada Health Act, ambulance services are not. They are provincially and territorially regulated and funded. As a result, persons receiving paramedic services may receive a bill for those services. Billing amounts are often dependent on the province or territory of citizenship for the patient. For example, ambulance services in Ontario are considered co-funded by that province's health insurance plan, so a resident of Ontario is billed for a lesser amount than is a nonresident.

It is helpful for paramedics to be familiar with any applicable fee structure and the means of collection for provision of the services in their jurisdiction. The ability of a patient to pay such a fee is generally not a consideration, as policies govern the collection of amounts owing after a call has been completed. At the time of a request for service, paramedics are expected to respond to the call. If a patient asks, he or she has the right to be informed about what fees they will be charged.

# DEATH AND RESUSCITATION ISSUES

Resuscitation related issues are complex and can raise a multitude of legal, ethical, and moral questions and debate. They have implications for paramedics with respect to withholding or stopping resuscitation, knowledge of advance directives, understanding organ donation, and death in the field.

## Death in the Field: Witholding or Stopping Resuscitation

### OBVIOUS AND LEGAL DEATH

Generally, paramedics should not attempt resuscitation in a setting of clinical death with obvious signs of nonviability, such as decapitation, transection of the body, gross rigor mortis or lividity, full body burn with charring of remains, decomposition, or extensive outpouring of cranial or visceral contents (see Chapter 4, *Mosby's Paramedic Textbook*).

In addition, if a physician licensed in the given province or territory of the occurrence is present and has legally pronounced death, resuscitative care should not be initiated. However, in all cases, thorough documentation of the specifics is still required.

Clinical death otherwise generally warrants resuscitative effort. The potential for receiving online medical direction to cease resuscitation efforts varies from jurisdiction to jurisdiction but is most commonly associated with the ACP scope of practice or higher. In other jurisdictions, PCPs may also have well defined Termination of Resuscitation guidelines.

## PRONOUNCEMENT OF DEATH

The paramedic must be familiar with local medical directives, policies, and regulation concerning procedures to be followed regarding whether or not to initiate resuscitation and when to cease efforts. This often depends on the ability of the paramedic to consult directly with a coroner or delegating Base Hospital Physician. For example, ACPs may, in consideration of the clinical history of a given case, make a phone call to a base hospital physician to receive a cease resuscitation order, also known as a field pronouncement or pronouncement of death by proxy. There is considerable variation from area to area. Where there are such guidelines, they are typically based upon criteria such as

- unwitnessed arrest, or confirmed down-time of greater than 30 minutes, or other predetermined length of time;
- no defibrillatory shocks having been given at any time, and patient is presently in a non-shockable rhythm; and
- no return of spontaneous circulation noted at any time during resuscitative efforts.

When making a determination of death, or that resuscitation efforts will/should be terminated after they have already begun, the paramedic must be familiar with the relevant legislation in his or her province or territory, including the required form of contact with the appropriate authorities. If invasive acts have been performed, such as intravenous therapy or endotracheal intubation, they should be left in place after death for the coroner's review. An inserted intravenous should be clamped off so it does not continue to run, but otherwise left in situ.

If family members are present, it is important to provide emotional support and empathy. They may have questions such as those related to transport and disposition of the body. Paramedics should be well versed on the requirements so they can assist relatives and friends of the deceased in a compassionate and empathetic manner.

## Do Not Resuscitate Orders and Advance Directives

Despite a growing support for and trend toward living wills, Do-Not-Resuscitate (DNR) orders and advance care directives, most EMS agencies in Canada have continued with the practice of mandating resuscitative interventions unless obvious death has been determined. Formal recognition of living wills, DNR orders, and advance directives have been a source of ethical conflict for many paramedics

faced with the desire to respect patient wishes but being precluded from doing so in many cases of death.

Gradually, however, there is a shift away from this historical approach to prehospital management of death, and many EMS systems are developing more humane policies that permit withholding or termination of resuscitation under specified circumstances. This is of particular importance when speaking of those paramedics who do not have the option of contacting a Base Hospital Physician to pronounce death; such is typically the case for PCPs.

In 2001, Canadian researchers published the results of a study designed to identify potential field criteria for predicting 100% nonsurvival when the presenting rhythm is asystole in a Basic Life Support-Defibrillation (BLS-D) system. They concluded that call response times of greater than 8 minutes and a presenting rhythm of asystole were 100% predictive of nonsurvival.[5] This study, among others in the late 1990s and early twenty-first century, including the much celebrated OPALS study (Ontario Prehospital Advanced Life Support Study), have merely added to the growing field of international literature and consensus pertaining to ethical termination of resuscitation efforts.[6]

There are now numerous examples of set policies governing the manner in which paramedics may withhold or terminate resuscitation for patients who have made their wishes known, or who have a substitute decision-maker (such as a relative with legal power of attorney) indicate that the patient would not have desired resuscitation. In some cases, particularly with institutional care settings for the elderly, specific forms have been created to assist paramedics with an ability to rapidly identify patients' wishes and be able to abide by them. A sample of such a form is provided in Figure 4–2 in Chapter 4 of *Mosby's Paramedic Textbook*, Third Edition.

However, the paramedic still has obligations to the dead or dying patient, even where there are provincial or territorial policies in place pertaining to withholding resuscitation. In the event of doubt, prudence dictates that the paramedic should err on the side of caution and initiate full resuscitation. Similarly, respecting a wish to withhold resuscitation when death occurs does not mean that the paramedic should withhold all treatment. A dying patient with an express wish not to be resuscitated is still entitled to care, such as splinting fractures, maintaining airway patency, or providing oxygen. The care provided in such instances is not specifically resuscitative and is unlikely to prolong life but is indicated to reduce pain and suffering and assists with maintaining patient comfort.

## Potential Organ Donation

The paramedic can play a key role in identifying potential organ donors who are dead or near death. Despite being one of the most prosperous nations in the world, Canada has a national organ donation rate that lags considerably behind other nations at only 14 donors per million population. At any given point in time, some estimates place as many as 4000 people waiting for organs across the country.[7] Often, signed organ donation cards are kept with provincial or territorial drivers' licences. Once found, this information should be communicated to receiving hospital staff so appropriate measures and safeguards can be initiated to preserve the donor status. Care must be taken, however, not to initiate transport of a body that has already been declared dead if it is prohibited by provincial legislation.

Vital donors are those who must still have a heartbeat and perfusion but are brain dead. They are typically, though not always, the victims of isolated severe head injuries, who are kept alive by ongoing life support. They may donate their hearts, lungs, kidneys, and pancreas. Nonvital donors are already clinically dead and usually in transit to the hospital. They can donate corneas, skin, bone, tendon, veins, and heart valves up to 24 hours following death.

When a potential donor is identified, the paramedic can play a vital role in increasing the probability of successful organ donation. If transport has begun or is permissible in accordance with local policies and procedures, effective airway management, oxygenation and ventilation, as well as cardiopulmonary resuscitation (CPR), if indicated, are essential. Any efforts to maintain organ perfusion and systemic blood pressure that are within the paramedic's scope of practice should be considered. If possible, even small measures, such as taping the patient's eyes shut to preserve natural lubrication around the cornea, is helpful.

Because of the geography of Canada and its demographics, not all regions (and not even all provinces or territories) may offer all types of transplantations. This may necessitate the movement of human tissue or organs that have been donated by an urgent ambulance transport to a central hospital, while another ambulance may be required to move the potential recipient from his or her location to the same location where the donated organ is destined. Usually, kidneys are transplanted into patients living in the same region as the donor, but as many as one-third of donated lungs, hearts, and livers are given to patients who live in another region of the country.[7] In this sense, air ambulance utilization often makes the difference in the success of organ donation.

## CRIME SCENE RESPONSIBILITIES

Paramedics often respond to calls that turn out to be crime scenes. In some cases, this information is known beforehand, so the responding crew can approach with caution. In other cases, it is only after arriving at a scene that a crew realizes that a crime has taken place, or worse, that they are in the middle of a dangerous situation. In any of these cases, paramedics should consider that they have three primary concerns when responding to a potential crime scene: (1) being aware of maintaining personal safety for paramedics and other responders; (2) focusing on providing proper patient care to any patient who may require it, and;

(3) preserving evidence and minimizing contamination of the scene to the extent possible.

The personal safety of paramedics is of paramount importance. When advised of possible violence, paramedics are well justified in waiting for police to arrive before entering a scene. In some jurisdictions, it may be possible to establish direct radio contact with the police. In others, information must be relayed among the police, paramedics, and their agency-specific dispatchers. In either case, effective communication is vital. Should a paramedic crew inadvertently find itself in the middle of a crime scene that is still dangerous, use of portable radios to immediately contact dispatch is indicated, and despite the potential of patients requiring medical attention, if the scene is not safe, paramedics should attempt to retreat to a safe location until the police arrive.

Once it is safe to enter a scene, patient care can begin, recognizing that emotions can run high in various responders. Professionalism and interagency cooperation are essential. It is a crime scene, and collection of evidence is a main police focus. However, patient care must also be respected, so it is expected that paramedics and the police find neutral ground in terms of minimizing contamination of evidence while providing care. Suggestions and tips for doing so can be found in Box 4–11, Chapter 4 of *Mosby's Paramedic Textbook*, Third Edition.

## WAYS TO MINIMIZE LEGAL RISK

A paramedic cannot avoid exposure to legal risk. Any disaffected patient can file or pursue a legal challenge alleging deficiencies in practice by the paramedic resulting in allegations of harm to the patient. Circumstances beyond the direct control of the paramedic establish and may increase his or her exposure to legal proceedings and legal risk. Claims of patient harm may also result in further, or derivative, claims by the family of the patient for associated harm to the family members. The issue for the practising paramedic is therefore not one of avoiding legal risk, but rather it is a question of minimizing legal risk and avoiding a successful legal challenge with respect to the conduct and practices of the paramedic in the particular circumstances.

There are several ways a paramedic can minimize legal risk and avoid the potential for a successful legal challenge to his or her practice. In its simplest sense, the best defence for a paramedic is prevention. Paramedic practice requires that they maintain practice competence and proficiency and the exercise of knowledge, skills, practices and judgment to meet the applicable legal and ethical framework for the standards and scope of practice reasonably expected of a paramedic in the care and transport of each patient. Those expectations include an awareness of appropriate conduct in general interactions with co-workers and members of the public, and of governing standards in dealing with patient situations and needs.

Overall there are four main ways a paramedic can minimize his or her legal risk. The first is to understand the sources of liability to avoid common pitfalls. The second is understanding and ensuring informed consent in all practice situations. The third is to maintain currency of professional practice in accordance with generally applicable standards of practice, including knowledge and applicability of medical directives, employer policies and procedures, legislative acts and regulations, and general ethical and legal guidelines for practice. Fourth, and perhaps the most important, is to recognize the need to maintain professional standards of documentation in order to have a clear and contemporaneous record of events. In summary, ensuring informed consent and patient confidentiality and knowing and meeting appropriate standards of practice, supported by clear, concise, and complete documentation are critical in defending allegations of negligence, incompetence, or misconduct.[8,9]

## Liability Insurance

Paramedics perform hazardous work such as driving at high speeds and in poor conditions and performing patient care procedures in less than ideal circumstances. In one study conducted over a 10-year period in a major urban centre, motor vehicle collisions involving an ambulance accounted for the majority (72%) of legal claims, and medical negligence claims were few but were the next largest cause of dollars lost (35%).[3]

In addition, paramedics perform more controlled medical acts than virtually all other allied healthcare disciplines. They also apply their knowledge and skills in the most challenging of environments—the out-of-hospital environment. Therefore, liability insurance is a necessity for all paramedics. However, in most cases, ambulance or paramedic services provide that insurance for their employees as Liability Insurance Risk Management is a core function of ambulance services. Some regulated healthcare professions require that their members carry their own malpractice insurance.

This may be particularly important to the paramedic in circumstances where ambulance services are provided by private interests that may no longer be in business when a legal claim is initiated. In that circumstance, the paramedic may incur legal defence costs not only in defending the matter but also in proceedings to force the former employer's insurer to recognize and meet its obligations with respect to vicarious liability, if applicable.

In addition to malpractice insurance, professional liability insurance, if available, is recommended where the paramedic may be subject to professional proceedings before his or her governing body. This is not an insurable risk, except to the extent of legal representation, which can be costly in any legal proceeding.

● ● ● 　## SUMMARY

- The legal system in Canada derives from two main historical sources of relevance: English Common Law and French Civil Law. English common law tradition is applied throughout Canada, except in Quebec, in all matters of private law (such as lawsuits), while similar matters in Quebec are dealt with under the Civil Code tradition. However, for public laws such as The Criminal Code, common law applies throughout Canada.
- Laws in Canada can be federal, provincial, or territorial. Statutes are acts, while Regulations provide structure and details about how laws are applied.
- Private law relates to matters of a private nature and interactions between people. Cases involving private law result in settlement, or withdrawal, or in court by way of a lawsuit.
- To safeguard against negative employment consequences, litigation, or criminal convictions, paramedics must be familiar with the relevant legislation and regulations governing employment and paramedic practice in their province or territory.
- Paramedics must be familiar with the mandatory reporting procedure and provincial or territorial requirements for mandatory or voluntary reporting of such things as suspected child abuse, elder abuse, sexual assault, domestic violence, gunshot wounds, animal bites, or certain infectious diseases.
- Civil lawsuits against paramedics or EMS agencies are usually brought about as a result of allegations of negligence due to a real or perceived failure to exercise the standard of care expected of a reasonable or prudent paramedic with similar training in similar circumstances.
- The best protection for individual paramedics and entire EMS organizations is threefold: (1) adequate training, policies, and procedures that ensure due diligence; (2) provision of patient care that is consistent with both well-defined and commonly accepted standards of practice; and (3) meeting the requirements of professional documentation.
- Maintenance of patient confidentiality is a critical to paramedic practice. Confidential information applies to verbal and written information and includes details such as medical history and patient care rendered, provincial health insurance card number, name, and address. Provincial acts and regulations prescribe the requirement, including exceptions to non-disclosure and the need for patient consent in all other circumstances.

- A patient deemed to be competent and who has reached the age of majority always has the right to give or refuse consent to treatment, unless there are legal processes in place to suspend this right. This right exists even if the decision made has serious consequences, provided the paramedic took diligent steps to advise the patient of these consequences and ensured that the patient understood the advice given.

- A competent patient has the right to decide what care to receive or refuse, as well as the right to choose to be transported or not.

- Legal complications related to consent include *abandonment* issues, *forcible confinement*, and *assault*. To avoid abandonment allegations, paramedics must be aware that legal obligations do not end until transfer of care has been achieved and that the transfer of care is to a person with a suitable scope of practice who will be able to maintain care needs.

- Resuscitation issues that affect paramedics include withholding or terminating resuscitation, advance directives, organ donation, and handling death in the field setting.

- The three issues of greatest importance to paramedics when attending to the scene of foul play or criminal wrong-doing include (1) being aware of maintaining personal safety, (2) focusing on providing proper patient care to any patient who may require it, and (3) preserving evidence and minimizing contamination of the scene to the extent possible.

- Patient care documentation must be clear, concise, accurate, legible, and complete and should be done in a timely fashion. In general, if it was not recorded, it is assumed not to have been done.

# WEBLINKS

Alberta College of Paramedics
www.collegeofparamedics.org
The Alberta College of Paramedics is a self-governing body under the Alberta Health Disciplines Act. This is a good site for information on paramedic self-regulation and to learn about requirements for professional status such as competence, safe practice, and ethical behaviour.

Canadian Legal Information Institute (CanLII)
www.canlii.org
CanLII is a not-for-profit organization initiated by the Federation of Law Societies of Canada. It is a primary source of Canadian law. Information of legislation relative to paramedic practice in all provinces and territories as well as legal commentaries can be found on this Web site.

Department of Justice Canada
www.canada.justice.gc.ca
This Web site will provide an additional source of Canadian statutes and regulations, with links to provincial and territorial law information.

Office of the Privacy Commissioner of Canada
http://www.privcom.gc.ca/information/comms_e.asp
This Web site provides links to all provincial/territorial privacy laws.

# REFERENCES

1. *The Quebec Charter of Human Rights and Freedoms*, Part 1, Section 2. (R.S.Q.C. -12). 2006. Available at http://www.cdpdj.qc.ca/en/commun/docs/charter.pdf. Accessed July 26, 2006.

2. Sneiderman B., Irvine J.C., Osborne P.H. *Canadian Medical Law: An Introduction for Physicians, Nurses and Other Health Care Professionals,* 3rd ed. Ottawa, Ont: Carswell; 1995.

3. Colwell CB, Pons P, Blanchet JH, Mangino C. Claims against a paramedic ambulance service: a ten-year experience. *J Emerg Med.* 1999;17(6):999–1002.

4. *Canadian Charter of Rights and Freedoms.* Part 1, Section 15. Available at http://laws.justice.gc.ca/en/charter/index.html. Accessed July 26, 2006.

5. Petrie, DA. De Maio V, Stiell I, Dreyer J, Martin M, O'Brien J. Factors affecting survival after prehospital asystolic cardiac arrest in a Basic Life Support-Defibrillation system. *Can J Emerg Med.* 2001;3(3): 186–192.

6. Stiell IG, Wells GA, Field B, et al. OPALS Study Group. Advanced cardiac life support in out-of-hospital cardiac arrest. *N Engl J Med.* 2004;351: 647–656.

7. London Health Sciences Centre Multi-Organ Transplant Program.

8. MacDonald RD, Schwartz B, Sawadsky BV, Verbeek R, Mazza C. A Canadian fellowship training program in emergency medical services. *Can J Emerg Med.* November 2005; 7(6):406–410.

9. Grant A, Ashman A. *A Nurse's Practical Guide to the Law.* Aurora, Ont: Professional Press/Canada Law Books Inc., 1997.

# APPENDIX A
# Emergency Drug Index
## CANADIAN SUPPLEMENT

The Emergency Drug Index is a list of commonly used medications in prehospital care; it is not intended to be a complete guide to all emergency medications. For additional drug information, consult other standard references or pharmacology textbooks. Drugs included in this index are not found in *Mosby's Paramedic Textbook* and have been included in this supplemental list at the request of professors of paramedicine from across Canada. The drugs are listed alphabetically by generic name. The trade name(s) are shown in parentheses.

Abciximab (Reopro)
Carboprost tromethamine (Hemabate)
Clopidogrel bisulphate (Plavix)
Dantrolene sodium (Dantrium)
Dimenhydrinate (Gravol)
Enoxaparin (Lovenox)

Milrinone lactate (Apo-milrinone)
Nitroprusside (Nipride)
Propofol (Diprovan)
Rocuronium bromide (Zemuron)
Salbutamol (Ventolin)
Tenecteplase recombinant (TNKase)

## Abciximab

### CLASS
Antithrombotic, antiplatelet, glycoprotein IIb/IIIa platelet inhibitors

### DESCRIPTION
Human–murine monoclonal antibody Fab fragment. It binds to glycoprotein IIb/IIIa receptor sites on platelets. It interferes with platelet membrane function by inhibiting fibrinogen binding and platelet-to-platelet interaction, thus inhibiting platelet aggregation.

### ONSET AND DURATION
Intravenous
Onset: >90% inhibition of platelet aggregation within 2 hr
Duration: Approximately 48 hr

### INDICATIONS
Acute myocardial infarction (AMI), but only as adjunctive therapy to percutaneous transluminal coronary angioplasty (PTCA). Use of this drug requires that partial thromboplastin (PT) be checked prior to administration. Therefore paramedics will likely see this drug used only when patients are transferred from a distant hospital to a cardiac centre for rescue angioplasty.

### CONTRAINDICATIONS
Hypersensitivity to abciximab or murine proteins
Active internal bleeding
History of cerebrovascular accident (CVA) within two years or of CVA with severe neurological deficits
Concomitant use of anticoagulant unless PT<1.2 times control
Thrombocytopenia (<100,000 cells/mL)
Recent major surgery or trauma
Intracranial neoplasm
Aneurysm
Severe hypertension
History of vasculitis
Use of dextran before or during PTCA

### ADVERSE REACTIONS
Hematological: intracranial or retroperitoneal bleeding, hematemesis, thrombocytopenia
CNS: dizziness, confusion
GI: nausea, vomiting
Respiratory: pneumonia, pleural effusion
Local: pain, edema

### DRUG INTERACTIONS
The following may increase bleeding: oral anticoagulants; low-molecular-weight heparins (LMWHs) such

as dalteparin and tinzaparin; heparin; NSAIDs; clopidogrel; dipyridamole; ticlopidine, dextran.

## HOW SUPPLIED
2 mg/mL in 5-mL vials

## DOSAGE AND ADMINISTRATION
0.25 mg/kg over 5 min followed by 10 mg/min for the next 12 hr

## SPECIAL CONSIDERATIONS
Pregnancy safety: Category C
Vial should not be shaken.
Drug should be discarded if opaque particles are seen.
Monitor for bleeding at all potential sites.

# Carboprost Tromethamine (Hemabate)

## CLASS
Prostaglandin, oxytocic, abortifacient

## DESCRIPTION
Synthetic analogue of naturally occurring prostaglandin $F_2$ alpha. It stimulates myometrial contractions of the gravid uterus similar in quality to those occurring during labour.

## ONSET AND DURATION
Intramuscular
Onset: 15 min, peak: 15–60 min
Duration: <4 hr

## INDICATIONS (PREHOSPITAL)
Control of refractory postpartum hemorrhage due to lack of uterine muscle tone

## CONTRAINDICATIONS
Hypersensitivity to carboprost tromethamine, sodium chloride, and benzyl alcohol (components of the preparation)
Active cardiac, pulmonary, renal, or hepatic disease
Acute pelvic inflammatory disease (PID)
Pregnancy, lactation

## ADVERSE REACTIONS
CNS: headache, paraesthesias, flushing, anxiety, weakness, syncope, dizziness
Respiratory: coughing, dyspnea
CV: hypotension, arrhythmias, chest pain
GI: vomiting, diarrhea, nausea
GU: endometritis, perforated uterus, uterine rupture, uterine/vaginal pain, incomplete abortion
Chills
Diaphoresis
Backache
Breast tenderness

Eye pain
Skin rash
Pyrexia

## DRUG INTERACTIONS
Oxytocin or other oxytocics
Alcohol (also an oxytocic)

## HOW SUPPLIED
0.25 mg/mL (or 250 µg/mL)

## DOSAGE AND ADMINISTRATION
Adult (postpartum hemorrhage): 0.25 mg (250 µg) deep IM, repeated every 15–90 min, up to maximum of 2 mg
Pediatric: N/A

## SPECIAL CONSIDERATIONS
Pregnancy safety: Category D

# Clopidogrel bisulphate (Plavix)

## CLASS
Adenosine diphosphate (ADP) receptor antagonist, antiplatelet agent

## DESCRIPTION
Blocks ADP receptors on platelets, thus inhibiting ADP-mediated activation of the glycoprotein GP IIb/IIIa complex. This helps prevent platelet aggregation.

## ONSET AND DURATION
PO
Onset: varies (peak: 75 min)
Duration: 3–4 hr

## INDICATIONS (PREHOSPITAL)
Chest pain consistent with cardiac ischemia or AMI.
Also proven to be of benefit in the treatment of acute or unstable angina to prevent progression to AMI
Prophylaxis in the prevention of stroke, AMI

## CONTRAINDICATIONS
Allergy to clopidogrel
Pregnancy, lactation
Caution: bleeding disorders, recent surgery, intracranial hemorrhage

## ADVERSE REACTIONS
CNS: headache, dizziness, weakness, syncope, flushing
CV: chest pain, edema, hypertension
Respiratory: upper respiratory infection (URI), dyspnea, bronchitis, rhinitis, cough
GI: nausea, dyspepsia, constipation, diarrhea, GI bleeding
Dermatological: skin rash, pruritus
Flu-like syndrome

Increased bleeding risk
Arthralgia
Back pain

## DRUG INTERACTIONS
Potential increased risk of bleeding with NSAIDs, warfarin, heparin, LMWH, glycoprotein inhibitors

## HOW SUPPLIED
75-mg tablets

## DOSAGE AND ADMINISTRATION
Adult: 300 mg PO loading dose (followed by 75 mg daily)
Pediatric: Safety not established

## SPECIAL CONSIDERATIONS
Pregnancy safety: Category B

# Dantrolene sodium (Dantrium)

## CLASS
Skeletal muscle relaxant–direct

## DESCRIPTION
Relaxes muscle at a site beyond the myoneural junction. It is unclear how dantrolene achieves muscle relaxation, but it is likely due to prevention of the release of calcium stores from the intracellular sarcoplasmic reticulum.

## ONSET AND DURATION
Intravenous
Onset: rapid
Duration: 6–8 hr

## INDICATIONS (PREHOSPITAL)
Malignant hyperthermia crisis
Preoperative or procedural prophylaxis (e.g., administration of general anaesthetics and depolarizing neuro-muscular blocking agents)
(PO) Muscle spasticity associated with stroke, MS, CP, spinal cord injury

## CONTRAINDICATIONS
Active hepatic disease
Spasticity used to sustain upright posture, to maintain balance in locomotion, or to gain or retain increased function
Lactation

## ADVERSE REACTIONS
CNS: drowsiness, dizziness, weakness, general malaise, fatigue, speech disturbance, seizure, headache, lightheadedness, visual disturbance, diplopia, alteration of taste, insomnia, mental depression, mental confusion, increased nervousness
CV: tachycardia, erratic BP, phlebitis, effusion with pericarditis

GI: diarrhea, constipation, GI bleeding, anorexia, dysphagia, gastric irritation, abdominal cramps, hepatitis
GU: increased urinary frequency, hematuria, crystalluria, difficult erection, urinary incontinence, nocturia, dysuria, urinary retention
Dermatological: abnormal hair growth, acne-like rash, pruritus, urticaria, eczematoid eruption, sweating, photosensitivity
Myalgia
Backache
Chills and fever
Feeling of suffocation

## DRUG INTERACTIONS
Alcohol and other CNS depressants: compounded CNS depression
Estrogens: increased risk of hepatotoxicity in women >35 years
Calcium channel blockers: increased risk of ventricular fibrillation and cardiovascular collapse

## HOW SUPPLIED
20 mg/70-mL vial (vial contains 20 mg dantrolene sodium and 3000 mg mannitol). Reconstitute with 60 mL sterile water.

## DOSAGE AND ADMINISTRATION
Adult: Initial bolus of 1 mg/kg and continue until signs and symptoms subside or to a maximum of 10 mg/kg IV.
Prophylactic dose: 2.5 mg/kg IV 1 hr before surgery, infused over 1 hr
Pediatric: Same as adult; however, safety for use in children <5 years is not established

## SPECIAL CONSIDERATIONS
Pregnancy safety: Category C
Adverse effects (e.g., decreased muscle tone) may last as long as 14 days

# Dimenhydrinate (Gravol)

## CLASS
Antiemetic

## DESCRIPTION
The precise action of dimenhydrinate is not known. However, it may exert its antiemetic action through central anticholinergic action. It is believed to depress vestibular stimulation and labyrinthine functions or associated neural pathways.

Note: 90% of dimenhydrinate's effect is antihistaminic and only 10% is actually antiemetic. For this reason, this drug is often abused as a sedative or hypnotic for sleep aid. Like most antihistamines, it causes drowsiness.

## ONSET AND DURATION

Intravenous
Onset: immediate
Duration: 3–6 hr
Intramuscular
Onset: 20–30 min
Duration: 3–6 hr

## INDICATIONS

Nausea or vomiting
Prophylaxis for nausea and vomiting associated with transport by land, sea, or air, narcotic administration, vertigo due to Ménière's disease, or altered labyrinthine function

## CONTRAINDICATIONS

Allergy or sensitivity to dimenhydrinate or diphenhydramine
Narrow-angle glaucoma
Prostatic hypertrophy

## ADVERSE REACTIONS

CNS: drowsiness, confusion, nervousness, restlessness, headache, dizziness, vertigo, lassitude, tingling, heaviness and weakness of hands, insomnia and excitement (especially in children), hallucinations, convulsions, death, blurred vision, diplopia
CV: hypotension, dysrhythmias, tachycardia
Respiratory: nasal congestion, chest tightness, thickening of bronchial secretions
GI: dyspepsia, anorexia, nausea, vomiting, diarrhea or constipation, dryness of mouth, nose, and throat
Dermatological: urticaria, drug rash, photosensitivity

## DRUG INTERACTIONS

Alcohol and other CNS depressants: worsen CNS depression
Tricyclic antidepressants: exacerbate anticholinergic effects

## HOW SUPPLIED

50 mg/mL

## DOSAGE AND ADMINISTRATION

Adult: 25–50 mg IM or IV
IV dimenhydrinate should be diluted ≥1:10 in NS or other compatible solution and administered over 3–10 min
May cause burning sensation if given too quickly
Pediatric: 6–8 years: 12.5–25 mg IM or IV
8–12 years: 25–50 mg IM or IV
>12 years: 50 mg IM or IV

## SPECIAL CONSIDERATIONS

Pregnancy safety: Category B
Give as a slow bolus or as an infusion—may cause burning sensation if administered too quickly.
Should not be given parenterally to neonates

# Enoxaparin (Lovenox), Dalteparin (Innohep), Tinzaparin (Fragmin)

## CLASS

Anticoagulant, LMWH

## DESCRIPTION

Thrombolytic drugs expose trapped thrombin in the process of breaking up the clot and paradoxically enhance the prothrombotic processes. This increases the risk of reocclusion of the coronary vessel. Thus, antithrombotic therapy is important to maintain vessel patency. Enoxaparin inhibits thrombus and clot formation by blocking factor Xa and factor IIa and preventing the formation of clots. It increases thrombin time (TT) and activated partial thromboplastin time (aPTT) by up to 1.8 times the control value.

Note: Although they are essentially the same, the three currently used LMWHs are assigned different names due to the application process. The makers of enoxaparin applied for and received government approval for use in angina and MI. The makers of tinzaparin applied for and received approval for use in deep-vein thrombosis (DVT) and pulmonary embolism (PE); the makers of dalteparin applied for and received approval for use in clot prophylaxis after orthopedic surgery.

## ONSET AND DURATION

Intravenous
Onset: rapid
Duration: 4.6 hr
Subcutaneous injection
Onset: 20–60 min
Duration: 4.6 hr

## INDICATIONS (PREHOSPITAL)

Adjunctive therapy for acute ST elevation MI (STEMI)

## CONTRAINDICATIONS

Hypersensitivity to enoxaparin, heparin, pork products
Severe thrombocytopenia
Uncontrolled bleeding

## ADVERSE REACTIONS

Hematological: hemorrhage, bruising, thrombocytopenia, hyperkalemia, hypersensitivity
Chills, fever
Pain
Urticaria
Asthma
Local irritation, hematoma, erythema at site of injection

## DRUG INTERACTIONS

Oral anticoagulants (clopidrogel, heparin), salicylates, penicillins, cephalosporins: increased bleeding tendencies.

Herbal products (garlic, ginger, ginkgo, feverfew, and horse chestnut): may also increase the risk of bleeding.

## HOW SUPPLIED (INJECTION)
30 mg/0.3 mL
40 mg/0.4 mL
60 mg/0.6 mL
80 mg/0.8 mL
Multidose vial: 300 mg/3 mL

## DOSAGE AND ADMINISTRATION
Adult: 0.5 mg/kg IV, followed by 1 mg/kg subsequent dose (follow local medical directive)
1 mg/kg SC bid
Pediatric: Safety not established

## SPECIAL CONSIDERATIONS
Pregnancy safety: Category B

# Milrinone lactate (Apo-milrinone)

## CLASS
Cardiotonic agent, inotropic agent, vasodilator

## DESCRIPTION
Positive inotropic effect (increases force of contraction of ventricles) by inhibiting cyclic-AMP phosphodiesterase; vasodilation by a direct relaxant effect on vascular smooth muscle.

## ONSET AND DURATION
Intravenous
Onset: Immediate
Duration: 2 hr

## INDICATIONS
Acute exacerbation of congestive heart failure (CHF)

## CONTRAINDICATIONS
Allergy to milrinone or bisulphites
Severe aortic or pulmonic valvular disease

## ADVERSE EFFECTS
CV: Ventricular or supraventricular dysrhythmias, hypotension, chest pain, angina
Hematological: thrombocytopenia, hypokalemia
Death

## DRUG INTERACTIONS
Disopyramide: may cause excessive hypotension.

## HOW SUPPLIED
1 mg/mL

## DOSAGE AND ADMINISTRATION
Adult: 50 µg/kg IV bolus loading dose over 10 min, followed by maintenance infusion of 0.375 to 0.75 µg/kg/min. Not to exceed a total of 1.13 mg/kg per day.
Note: Should be diluted with 180 mL per 20-mg vial (20 mL) using 0.45% or 0.9% sodium chloride or 5% dextrose to yield a 100 µg/mL solution.
Pediatric: Not recommended

## SPECIAL CONSIDERATIONS
Pregnancy safety: Category C
Precipitates if given in the same intravenous line as furosemide
Also incompatible with procainamide

# Nitroprusside (Nipride)

## CLASS
Antihypertensive, vasodilator

## DESCRIPTION
Acts directly on vascular smooth muscle by interfering with calcium influx into cells and with release of intracellular calcium stores. This causes arterial and venous vasodilation and reduction of blood pressure. Reflex tachycardia may occur in response to hypotensive effect.

## ONSET AND DURATION
IV infusion
Onset: 1–2 min
Duration: 1–10 min

## INDICATIONS
Hypertensive crisis for immediate reduction of BP
Acute CHF

## CONTRAINDICATIONS
Compensatory hypertension

## ADVERSE REACTIONS
CNS: apprehension, headache, restlessness, muscle twitching, dizziness
CV: retrosternal pressure, dysrhythmias, bradycardia, tachycardia
GI: nausea, vomiting, abdominal pain
Hematological: methemoglobinemia, antiplatelet effects
Dermatological: diaphoresis, flushing
Endocrine: hypothyroidism
Local: irritation at injection site
Cyanide toxicity (seen in overdose): increasing tolerance to drug and metabolic acidosis are early signs, followed by dyspnea, headache, vomiting, dizziness, ataxia, loss of consciousness, imperceptible pulse, absent reflexes,

widely dilated pupils, pink colour, distant heart sounds, shallow breathing

## DRUG INTERACTIONS
No clinically significant interactions, although it should not be used concurrently with nitroglycerin drip due to the high risk of sudden hypotension

Should not be mixed with any other drug or with any solution other than D5W. Note that IV tubing should be wrapped in foil as the solution is light sensitive

## HOW SUPPLIED
50-mg vial (powder that requires reconstitution with sterile water or D5W).

## DOSAGE AND ADMINISTRATION
Adult: 0.5 to 10 µg/kg/min (average of 3 µg/kg/min). Must be mixed with D5W for infusion.
Pediatric: Same as adult

## SPECIAL CONSIDERATIONS
Pregnancy safety: Category C
Elderly patients may be more susceptible to hypotensive effects.
Drug should be used within 4 hr of being reconstituted.

# Propofol (Diprovan)

## CLASS
Induction agent, general anaesthetic, sedative-hypnotic

## DESCRIPTION
The mechanism of action of propofol is unclear; however, it is believed to positively modulate the inhibitory function of gama-aminobutyric acid (GABA). When GABA interacts with its receptor in the CNS, adjacent chloride channels open, allowing an influx of the negatively charged chloride ion into the cell, which results in sedation. Propofol affects a different GABA subtype than do benzodiazepines.

## ONSET AND DURATION
Intravenous
Onset: ≤40–60 sec
Duration: 6–10 min

## INDICATIONS
Induction and maintenance of anaesthesia
Conscious sedation, procedural sedation

## CONTRAINDICATIONS
Hypersensitivity to propofol or propofol emulsion (soya bean oil, egg, etc.)
Obstetrical procedures
Increased intracranial pressure (ICP)
Lactation

Age <3 years
Use with caution in patients with severe cardiac or respiratory disorders or history of seizures.

## ADVERSE REACTIONS
Respiratory: cough, upper airway obstruction, apnea, hypoventilation, and dyspnea
Note: A rapid bolus injection can result in significant cardiorespiratory depression, including hypotension, apnea, airway obstruction, and oxygen desaturation.

## DRUG INTERACTIONS
Alfentanil is potentiated.

## HOW SUPPLIED
200 mg in 20 mL (10 mg/mL) given undiluted

## DOSAGE AND ADMINISTRATION
Adult: 2–2.5 mg/kg IV q 10 min until induction onset (rate of injection approx 10 mg/sec). Conscious sedation protocols may vary by region or hospital; however, one suggested protocol calls for the same dose per kg but starting with a 20–30 mg bolus, followed by 10–20 mg every 1–2 min until satisfactory anaesthesia is achieved. 10 mg/sec is high for conscious sedation and poses a high risk of apnea.
Geriatric: 1–1.5 mg/kg IV q 10 min until induction onset
Pediatric (≥3 years): 125–300 µg/min IV
Conscious sedation: 5 µg/kg/min for at least 5 min. May increase to 5–10µg/kg/min until desired sedation is achieved.

## SPECIAL CONSIDERATIONS
Pregnancy safety: Category B
Associated with increased incidence of bacteremia: strict aseptic technique required
Note: Excess must be discarded as there is a very high risk of sepsis due to the egg content. This drug has a very high contamination rate if not handled properly.
Should not be administered in same IV line as other medication

# Rocuronium Bromide (Zemuron)

## CLASS
Nondepolarizing neuromuscular blocking agent, paralytic

## DESCRIPTION
Competes for cholinergic receptors at the motor endplates. In so doing, nondepolarizing neuromuscular blocking agents prevent acetylcholine from reaching skeletal muscles to allow for normal muscle tone and contraction. This results in paralysis of skeletal muscles.

## ONSET AND DURATION
Intravenous
Onset: <2 min
Duration: 20–30 min

## INDICATIONS
To facilitate endotracheal intubation
To provide skeletal muscle relaxation during surgery
To facilitate mechanical ventilation in intubated, critically ill, or injured patients

## CONTRAINDICATIONS
Known hypersensitivity to rocuronium bromide
Caution: myasthenia gravis

## ADVERSE EFFECTS
CV: bradycardia or tachycardia, hypertension or hypotension
Respiratory: bronchospasm, anaphylaxis
Rash
Hypothermia
Corneal ulceration
Excessive salivation

## DRUG INTERACTIONS
Aminoglycosides, clindamycin, inhaled anaesthetics, amphotericin B, quinidine, magnesium salts: increased neuromuscular blocking effect. Blocking effects are also increased in the presence of hypokalemia.
Steroids: possible increased risk of myopathy
Anticonvulsants: possible decreased effect of rocuronium
Phenytoin and carbamazepine: possible decreased effect or shortened duration

## HOW SUPPLIED
10 mg/mL (50 mg in 5 mL)

## DOSAGE AND ADMINISTRATION
Adult: 0.6–1.2 mg/kg (0.6 mg/kg usually sufficient; 1 mg/kg dose often used for simplicity)
Pediatric: 0.6 mg/kg

## SPECIAL CONSIDERATIONS
Pregnancy safety: Category C
Not recommended for cesarean section patients

# Salbutamol (Ventolin)

## CLASS
Sympathomimetic, bronchodilator, beta$_2$ agonist

## DESCRIPTION
Salbutamol is a sympathomimetic that is selective for beta$_2$ adrenergic receptors. It relaxes the smooth muscles of the bronchial tree, likely through stimulation of adenyl cyclase, resulting in increased levels of cyclic-AMP within cells. This results in a decrease in influx of calcium ions into the cells and consequent inhibition of smooth muscle contraction. Salbutamol also causes vasodilation of peripheral vasculature. Repeating doses of salbutamol increases beta$_1$ effects and may cause tachycardia and dysrhythmias.

## ONSET AND DURATION
Onset: 5–15 min after inhalation
Duration: 3–4 hr after inhalation

## INDICATIONS
Relief of bronchospasm in patients with reversible obstructive airway disease
Prevention of exercise-induced bronchospasm
Also useful for hyperkalemic patients with renal failure as it causes increased cellular uptake of K+. It is considered a temporary adjunct, along with insulin, glucose, calcium, and bicarbonate, in the treatment of life-threatening hyperkalemia.

## CONTRAINDICATIONS
Prior hypersensitivity reaction to salbutamol
Cardiac dysrhythmias associated with tachycardia
Known hypokalemia
Use with caution in patients with diabetes mellitus, hyperthyroidism, prostatic hypertrophy, seizure disorder, or cardiovascular disorder.

## ADVERSE REACTIONS
## (USUALLY DOSE RELATED)
CNS: Restlessness, apprehension, dizziness
CV: palpitations, tachycardia, dysrhythmias

## DRUG INTERACTIONS
Other sympathomimetics may exacerbate adverse cardiovascular effects.
Antidepressants may potentiate vasodilation effects.
Beta blockers may antagonize salbutamol.
Salbutamol may potentiate diuretic-induced hypokalemia.

## HOW SUPPLIED
Metered dose inhaler (MDI): 100 µg/metered spray
Solution for nebulization: 0.5% (5 mg/mL); 0.083% (2.5 mg) in 2.5- and 5-mL nebules

## DOSAGE AND ADMINISTRATION
Acute bronchial asthma
Adult: MDI: 1 inhalation (100 µg) q4 breaths, repeat prn as per local medical directives.
Solution: 5 mg, administer over 5–15 min and repeat prn as per local medical directives.
Pediatric: MDI: 1 inhalation (100 µg) q4 breaths, repeat prn as per local medical directives.
Solution: 2.5 mg, administer over 5–15 min and repeat prn as per local medical directives.

## SPECIAL CONSIDERATIONS

Pregnancy safety: Category C

May precipitate angina pectoris and dysrhythmias

MDI may be preferable in the presence of a febrile respiratory illness to reduce the paramedic's risk of exposure to droplets.

# Tenecteplase recombinant (TNKase)

## CLASS

Thrombolytic agent

## DESCRIPTION

Tenecteplase is a modified form of human tissue plasminogen activator (tPA) that binds to fibrin and converts plasminogen to plasmin. Plasmin lyses the clot by breaking down the fibrinogen and fibrin contained in a clot. TNKase has a 14-fold greater fibrin specificity than alteplase and a longer half-life.

## ONSET AND DURATION

Intravenous

Onset: rapid

Duration: 90–130 min half-life

## INDICATIONS

Acute STEMI or new-onset left-bundle branch block (LBBB) within 12 hr (ideally <6 hr) of symptom onset. In order to qualify for thrombolytics, a patient must have at least 30 min of chest pain and either 1 mm of ST elevation in two contiguous limb leads or 2 mm ST elevation in 2 contiguous precordial leads. In all other patients, the risks outweigh the benefits.

## CONTRAINDICATIONS

Active internal bleeding

History of CVA

Intracranial or intraspinal surgery within 2 mo

Intracranial neoplasm

Arteriovenous malformation or aneurysm

Known bleeding diathesis

Severe uncontrolled hypertension

Relative contraindications: There are many relative contraindications, including current use of anticoagulants with INR >2–3, prolonged CPR >10 min, recent surgery <3 wk, or recent internal bleeding. The clinician should consult with an appropriate reference and carefully weigh the risk-to-benefit ratio.

## ADVERSE REACTIONS

Hematological: major bleeding, hematoma, GI bleeding, bleeding at puncture site(s), hematuria, epistaxis

## DRUG INTERACTIONS

Anticoagulants and drugs that alter platelet function (such as acetylsalicylic acid, dipyridamole, and GP IIb/IIIa inhibitors) may increase the risk of bleeding if administered prior to, during, or after TNKase therapy.

## HOW SUPPLIED

50-mg vial

## DOSAGE AND ADMINISTRATION

Adult:

30 mg for patients <60 kg

35 mg for patients 60–70 kg

40 mg for patients 70–80 kg

45 mg for patients 80–90 kg

50 mg for patients >90 kg

Pediatric: Safety not established

## SPECIAL CONSIDERATIONS

Pregnancy safety: Category C

In the ASSENT-2 trial, the rates of intracranial hemorrhage were 0.4% in patients <65, 1.6% in patients aged 65–74, and 1.7% in patients >75 years.

After administration, avoid unnecessary injections or other invasive procedures that may be a source of bleeding.

Monitor for signs and symptoms of acute bleeding.

# APPENDIX B
# Canadian Triage Acuity Scale

## INTRODUCTION

The Canadian Triage and Acuity Scale (CTAS) was developed to improve triage in Canadian emergency departments (EDs). CTAS is used to assign a level of severity of illness to patients, which is expected to correlate accurately with the urgency of the patient's need for care. CTAS has since been adapted in many EMS systems so that hospital EDs and paramedics in the field share a common triage system and terminology. The intent is to identify the patient's need for care prior to arrival at the hospital.

CTAS is based on the patient's presenting complaint, specific modifiers, and, in the case of prehospital care, the primary problem. Other factors come into play in determining the patient's acuity level. These include the patient's appearance, vital signs, pain severity, mechanism of injury, and associated symptoms or secondary modifiers. The patient is the focus of this triage system. The triage category provides a guideline for the optimal time to medical intervention within the hospital and the time interval for reassessments for those waiting to be seen.

The CTAS scale has five levels of severity, with the highest priority being level 1, resuscitation and the lowest priority level 5, nonurgent.

1. Level 1, resuscitation
2. Level 2, emergent
3. Level 3, urgent
4. Level 4, less urgent
5. Level 5, nonurgent

## APPLYING THE CTAS SCALE IN THE PREHOSPITAL SETTING

The same CTAS acuity scale applied in the ED is applied by paramedics in the field. The scale is applied *at the time of departure from the scene*, and the level of acuity is based on the patient's condition at that time. The assignment of the acuity level is based not only on the paramedic's initial assessment but also on examination findings, patient response to treatment, and the patient's status on departure.

The CTAS is applied at the time of departure from the scene and the level of acuity is based on the patient's condition at that time.

This assessment is not static and can be reapplied during transport. A change in patient status may require a change in acuity level assignment, with notification of the ED or the dispatcher of the change. The return priority codes (codes assigned after the paramedic crew has responded to the call) used by paramedics, although related to acuity, refer to the following:

- The urgency of a response or transport.
- Other use of an ambulance when a patient is not carried.

The radio patch identifying the return priority also contains the assigned CTAS acuity level. This standardizes the terminology for patients being transported to the hospital.

## Benefits of Using CTAS Acuity Scale in the Prehospital Setting

1. Having a common language improves communication among the field, the ED, and the dispatcher.
2. The scale helps hospital personnel understand the needs of patients coming to the ED and decide in advance what resources will be required.
3. The scale helps determine patient destination based on patient need and on the resources available.
4. The scale can be used to help hospitals with planning by tracking the types of patients arriving at EDs by ambulance over time.

## Assigning a CTAS Acuity Level to Prehospital Patients

**Rule 1: Assign the patient's acuity level at the time of departure from scene.** This level may be different from the level at the initial assessment due to treatment given or spontaneous change in the patient. For example, a patient has chest pain on arrival but subsequently has a cardiac arrest. This patient may have been a level 2 initially but clearly at departure is a level 1 requiring ongoing resuscitation.

**Rule 2: When taking into consideration the patient's response to treatment, assign an acuity level no more than 2 levels below the pretreatment acuity.** The patient could deteriorate again during transport.

**Rule 3: If the patient's condition deteriorates, notify the hospital of the change in the patient's status and acuity level.**

## Patient Priority in the Determination of Transport Destination

As discussed in Chapters 1 and 3, the destination decision is often made in consultation with the dispatcher and in accordance with local, provincial, or territorial policies. This decision may take the following into account:

1. The availability of helicopter response and transportation.
2. Specific patient needs, which may suggest a unit with a specialty, such as trauma, burns, strokes, percutaneous coronary intervention (PCI), pediatrics, or obstetrics.
3. The assigned CTAS level:
   - level 1—closest facility.
   - level 2—closest suitable facility, based on communication between paramedics, dispatch, and the receiving ED.
   - level 3, 4, 5—most available facility, based on communication between the dispatcher and the receiving ED. At these lower acuity levels, the decision may also take into consideration the patient's wishes.

While the final destination decision rests with the dispatch centre and your communications officer (CO), the above list serves as a guide for paramedics. Certainly, patients designated as level 1 are the highest priority and need to be transported to the nearest facility immediately.

With lower-acuity patients, hospitals' capacity to accept further patients may influence the decision. It is here that communication between the paramedics and the dispatcher and between the dispatcher and hospitals becomes essential. Dispatchers are often in regular contact with EDs and are updated on their ability to take patients. Assignment of CTAS levels better communicates the needs of the patient.

## Paramedic Patching

The patient's status is communicated to hospitals through the patch. Where CTAS is used, all patches should state the patient's age and sex, the CTAS acuity level, and the chief complaint or primary problem. Pertinent positive and negative findings should also be included, along with treatment and response. The estimated time of arrival (ETA) is also stated. Remember that patches for transport should be focused and brief. Thus, the components of the patch are

1. patient age and sex,
2. CTAS acuity level,
3. chief complaint,
4. abnormal findings and abnormal vital signs,
5. treatment given and response, and
6. ETA.

## CTAS CATEGORY DEFINITIONS AND PRESENTING COMPLAINTS

Each acuity level in CTAS is defined to give a better understanding of the types of problems that are encountered in each triage level. The assignment of the acuity level is based primarily on the chief complaint and first-order modifiers. The revised CTAS identifies common chief complaints, which in themselves often define the level of acuity. However, some chief complaints have many different acuity levels that are better defined by applying first-order modifiers and, if necessary, second-order modifiers. The first-order modifiers are vital signs, pain scales, and mechanism of injury.

However, paramedics are always encouraged to use their assessment skills, experience, and instinct to "up triage" a patient. If the facts and CTAS definitions suggest a lower acuity but your instinct tells you the patient needs immediate help, trust it. Remember, "If they look sick, then they probably are." However, the converse does not hold. Do *not* rely on your instinct to "down triage" to a lower acuity level when the facts suggest a more serious problem. For example, if a patient says she has chest pain that suggests a cardiac cause but she looks well, take the more serious possibilities first, assign a level 2, and allow the emergency physicians to determine the exact nature of the problem.

## Pain Scales

Pain is one of the first-order modifiers used to determine CTAS levels. The most common way to assess pain is to ask the patient to give the pain a number on a scale from 1 to 10, with 10 being the worst pain the person has ever experienced. Pain scoring high on the scale is assigned a higher level because of the need for pain relief. However, pain scales are difficult to use in assigning a level of acuity because of their subjective nature. When a patient claims to have a pain of 8–10/10 but does not appear to be in distress and does not have the signs you would expect to see, it is helpful to ask about the person's most painful previous experience. The first pain anyone has is by definition a 10 on the scale! If a patient is comparing the current pain with a previous experience of childbirth, a broken bone, renal colic, migraine, or other conditions expected to cause severe pain, this may help you decide which triage level is appropriate. If a child or elderly person is unable to verbally score the pain but is thought to have severe pain, consider the pain as 8–10/10. Chronic pain and recurring pain are assigned lower acuity than first-time pain of the same intensity.

## CTAS Level 1—Resuscitation

CTAS level 1 conditions include threats to life or limb (or imminent risk of deterioration) requiring immediate, aggressive interventions. These patients have a problem with their ABCs requiring immediate or continuing treatment *and* aggressive or resuscitative efforts *immediately* upon arrival at the ED. These patients are always transported to hospital with flashing lights and sirens on. The hospital needs to be informed of the CTAS level, pertinent patient information, and ETA.

**CTAS 1 guideline for time to physician in the ED is immediate.**

The following are the usual presentations of level 1.

## ARREST

Cardiac or pulmonary arrest, prearrest, and postarrest indicate level 1. This includes patients with *unstable* vital signs, such as confusion, agitation, decreased level of awareness (LOA), mottling and cold extremities, marked pallor, and markedly decreased $O_2$ saturation.

## MAJOR TRAUMA

Severe injury of any single body system is a level 1 emergency, as is multiple system injury. The following are indicators of major trauma:

- Head injury with GCS<10 or spinal injury with neurological deficit.
- Severe burns (>25% total body surface area or airway problems).
- Chest or abdominal injury with any of the following:
  - Hypotension and tachycardia, usually with severe pain (pain scale 8–10/10)
  - Respiratory distress with abnormal rate, volume, or decreased air entry
  - Altered mental state suggesting hypoxemia or hypoperfusion
  - Major trauma to a limb with neurovascular compromise.

## SHOCK STATES

These include conditions that create an imbalance between oxygen delivery (e.g., cardiogenic, pulmonary, blood loss, and third space loss) and demand or utilization (i.e., sepsis syndrome). Patients have hypotension and/or tachycardia, or possibly bradycardia in advanced prearrest situations. Shock states include all types of cardiogenic shock, pulmonary edema, sepsis, acute blood loss, severe burns, and anaphylaxis.

## UNCONSCIOUSNESS

Unconsciousness is indicated by a GCS <10 or acute decreased LOA requiring airway protection, support, or assisted ventilation. Examples are intoxication, overdose, central nervous system (CNS) events, metabolic disturbances, and active seizures.

Hypoglycemia is a rapidly reversible problem, which should be ascertained with glucometer screening tests and rapidly treated with IV glucose or SC/IM glucagon. Patients often respond before transport and may be given a lower acuity rating at departure.

## SEVERE RESPIRATORY DISTRESS

There are many causes for severe respiratory distress, such as CHF, pneumothorax, and near-death asthma. The latter is characterized by inability to speak, cyanosis, lethargy or confusion, tachycardia or bradycardia, $O_2$ saturation <90%, and exacerbations of chronic obstructive pulmonary disease (COPD).

## PREGNANCY

Any third-trimester pregnancy with vaginal bleeding is potentially life threatening for both the mother and the fetus (because of the risk of placenta previa or abruptio placentae). Patients in labour where any part of the fetus is showing should also be considered level 1.

# CTAS Level 2—Emergent

CTAS Level 2 conditions are a *potential* threat to life, limb, or function, requiring rapid medical intervention or controlled acts. These patients have serious illness or injury and have the potential for further deterioration that may then require resuscitation. They need prompt treatment to stabilize developing problems and treat acute conditions. These patients have often had controlled acts applied in the field but require further rapid intervention and treatment.

Level 2 patients have the potential for deterioration requiring aggressive measures. These patients are most often transported to hospital with lights and sirens. The hospital needs to be informed of the CTAS level, pertinent patient information, and ETA.

**CTAS 2 guideline for time to physician in the ED is ≤15 minutes**.

The following are the usual presentations.

## ALTERED MENTAL STATE

Altered mental status can take the form of cognitive deficits, agitation, lethargy, and confusion. Patients with GCS ≤13 fall into this level. Mental status changes may be caused by inflammatory, ischemic, or traumatic incidents, infections, poisoning, drug effects, and metabolic disorders. In infants, irritability and poor feeding are signs of altered mental status and could represent serious bacterial infection or dehydration.

## HEAD INJURY

This problem appears in several triage levels. Patients at high risk require a physician assessment within 15 minutes of arrival to determine the need for airway protection, computed tomography (CT) scanning, or neurosurgical intervention. These patients often have a persisting or declining altered mental state (GCS ≤13).

Loss of consciousness (LOC) ≥5 minutes, confusion, and severe headache with nausea or vomiting are present. Details regarding the time of impact, mechanism of injury, onset and severity of symptoms, and changes over time are very important and should be taken into account in assigning the level.

## SEVERE TRAUMA

These patients may have high-risk mechanisms of injury and either severe single system involvement or multiple system involvement with less severe signs and symptoms in each. Generally, physical assessment reveals severe pain (8–10/10) and abnormal vital signs, without signs of hypoperfusion. These patients may exhibit tachycardia only but are potentially unstable.

## NEONATES

Children ≤7 days are at risk for hyperbilirubinemia, undiagnosed congenital heart abnormalities, and sepsis. The signs of serious problems may be very subtle, from not feeding well to being less active or simply "not the same." Parental anxiety is often very high, and these patients should be assigned level 2.

## EYE PAIN

Chemical exposures (acid or alkali) cause severe pain (8–10/10) and blurred vision. The seriousness of these injuries puts them at level 2. Other severe painful conditions with associated visual loss such as glaucoma and iritis, also require prompt emergency assessment. Corneal foreign bodies and arc-weld injuries can often be assigned level 3.

## CHEST PAIN

This is one of the most difficult presenting complaints to assess. Cardiac ischemia presents in so many ways that paramedics often cannot reach a definite conclusion. Patients with nontraumatic visceral pain are most likely to have coronary ischemia (AMI, unstable angina). Careful documentation is needed of the activity at the onset, the duration of each episode, the character, the site, the radiation, associated symptoms, aggravating and alleviating factors, and risk profile. All these elements influence the prediction of significant coronary disease. This level includes all patients who meet the criteria for ASA or nitroglycerin (NTG), with or without IV access. Even patients who get relief from NTG should remain at level 2.

Sudden sharp pains can be associated with chest wall problems but can also be due to pulmonary embolus, aortic dissection, pneumothorax, pneumonia, or other serious problems. These pains are usually severe, sudden, and persistent or are associated with other symptoms such as shortness of breath (SOB) and syncope or presyncope. Often significant risk factors are present. Sharp pains that are not severe or that are easily reproduced by palpation or aggravated by cough, deep breathing, or movement can be assigned level 3 or 4 if the patient has normal vital signs.

## OVERDOSE

Patients who have taken intentional overdoses are particularly unreliable in reporting which agents they have ingested and how much. These patients require early physician assessment or advice on the need for toxic screening, monitoring, treatment to prevent absorption and enhance elimination, or administration of antidotes. Patients with any signs of significant toxicity (altered mental state, abnormal vital signs) should be assigned level 1.

## ABDOMINAL PAIN

Pain severity alone cannot predict whether serious surgical or medical conditions are present. Patients with visceral pain (constant ache, pressure, burning, squeezing), associated symptoms (nausea, vomiting, sweating, radiation, bump, or reverberating pain) and abnormal vital signs (e.g., hypertension, hypotension, tachycardia, fever) are much more likely to have serious problems that require prompt investigation, treatment, or pain relief. They should be assigned level 2. Generally, the physical assessment will reveal severe pain (8–10/10) and abnormal vital signs without signs of hypoperfusion.

Crampy, intermittent, or sharp, brief pains with lower pain scores and without vital sign abnormalities may be assigned level 3. There is significant overlap between benign conditions and catastrophes such as ruptured abdominal aortic aneurysm (AAA) (age >50), ectopic pregnancy (females 12–50), perforated viscus, bowel obstruction, and ascending cholangitis. Therefore any severe (8–10/10) or very sudden abdominal pain should be treated as an emergency.

## GASTROINTESTINAL BLEEDING

Upper gastrointestinal (GI) sources of bleeding are more likely to cause instability. Vomiting gross blood, coffee-ground emesis, and melena are typical of upper GI sources. Maroon stool, dark blood, or bright red blood can also be from upper GI sources but are more likely to be lower gastrointestinal. The source is not as important as how to deal with the patient with hemodynamic instability. One set of normal vital signs does not guarantee hemodynamic stability. These patients present with abnormal vital signs without signs of hypoperfusion.

## CEREBROVASCULAR ACCIDENT

Patients with *acute* onset of major neurological deficits suggestive of stroke may require airway protection or emergent CT scanning to determine criteria for thrombolysis, anticoagulation, or neurosurgical intervention. If the time of onset of symptoms is <3 hours, then time to CT scanning is a critical element in some treatment strategies.

## ASTHMA

Patients with moderate dyspnea, speaking in short sentences with some indrawing can be assigned level 2. Patients too short of breath to speak, with cyanosis or altered mental status, are level 1.

In children, particularly those under age 6, clinical features and $O_2$ saturation are used to estimate severity.

## DYSPNEA

Depending on the age, previous history, and physical assessment, you may not be able to distinguish among asthma, COPD, CHF, pulmonary embolism (PE), pneumothorax, pneumonia, croup, epiglottitis, anaphylaxis, and a combination of problems. Onset, duration and severity of symptoms, vital signs, and auscultation of the chest are used to assess severity.

## ANAPHYLAXIS

Severe allergic reactions can deteriorate rapidly. Patients with a history of asthma are at particularly high risk of death. Suspect problems if there are any respiratory symptoms (wheezing, SOB) or complaints of tightness or swelling in the throat. Patients in anaphylactic *shock* should be level 1.

## VAGINAL BLEEDING OR ACUTE PELVIC OR LOWER ABDOMINAL PAIN

Women with vaginal bleeding and/or acute lower abdominal pain (8–10/10) should be assessed for the possibility of ectopic pregnancy or other serious problems associated with pregnancy. These patients have abnormal vital signs without signs of hypoperfusion.

## PREGNANCY

Patients who may be in labour, with contractions as frequent as every 2 minutes, should be assigned level 2. Postdelivery patients are also level 2, unless there is maternal or neonatal distress, in which case they should be assigned level 1.

## SERIOUS INFECTIONS

Patients with serious bacterial infections or sepsis syndrome usually appear unwell and will have an abnormality in one or more physical signs such as mental state, vital signs, or O₂ saturation. A history of fever or chills with rigors should be elicited. (Rigor is a shaking episode that the patient cannot control.) Purpuric skin rashes with nonblanching spots and petechiae may be associated with meningitis.

## FEVER IN YOUNG INFANTS

Any fever (temperature ≥38°C) is of concern in infants under 3 months. This is often learned from the history given by the parent. The risk of a serious bacterial infection is much higher in young infants.

## FEVER IN CHILDREN OF ANY AGE

Fever and signs of lethargy (no energy, lying around, not active, listless) should lead you to consider serious bacterial illnesses such as meningitis.

## CHILDREN WITH LETHARGY

Lethargy, poor feeding, and vomiting, with or without a fever, may indicate serious illness.

## VOMITING AND DIARRHEA

Vomiting and diarrhea become an emergency if there are signs suggesting dehydration, particularly in association with abnormal vital signs. Tachycardia is the most common finding. Hypotension is a late finding that would require fluid resuscitation, thereby putting the child at level 1.

## ACUTE PSYCHOSIS OR EXTREME AGITATION

These patients may be suffering from metabolic disturbances, poisoning, substance abuse, or other organic problems. Vital signs, physical assessment, and history from other healthcare providers, witnesses, caregivers, family, or friends will often allow identification of those at risk from a medical perspective (e.g., overdose, CNS events, hypoglycemia). Patients requiring close supervision are level 2.

Risk of imminent harm to self or others or uncontrollable behaviour indicates level 1.

## DIABETES

Medical alert bracelets, history from others, physical assessment, vital signs, and glucose testing are all useful in identifying diabetics with hyper- or hypoglycemia. Diaphoresis and/or altered mental state are typical of hypoglycemia. Altered mental state, blurred vision, fever, vomiting, abnormal pulse, and rapid, deep respirations are more typical of hyperglycemia with or without diabetic ketoacidosis. Patients who are given glucagon or intravenous glucose and then become alert and responsive do not need to be designated level 2.

## PAIN IN THE FLANK, ABDOMEN, OR GROIN

Patients with renal colic (kidney stones) typically have very severe pain (8–10/10) within the flank, abdomen, groin, or testes. Nausea and sweating are common, but it is usually the severity of pain (with or without a prior history) that alerts care providers to the primary problem. A diagnosis of AAA has sometimes been missed or delayed because of some overlapping features in the history and physical presentation.

## HEADACHE

This presenting complaint appears in multiple triage levels. There are significant concerns about delays in diagnosing CNS catastrophes (subarachnoid, epidural, or subdural bleeding, meningitis, or encephalitis), which may have several overlapping features with migraine. Patients with migraines no different from usual can be assigned level 3. Key questions are activity at the time of onset, the suddenness of onset, neck symptoms, nausea or vomiting, and mental status. It is important to establish what a patient means by a "sudden pain." The critical question is how long it took to attain maximum intensity. Pains that are at their worst the moment they start ("like someone hit me with a two-by-four," or like a "thunderclap") or within a few seconds are almost always serious. Pains that get worse over a period of 5–30 minutes are typical of migraine.

## ABUSE, NEGLECT, OR ASSAULT

Patients who have experienced abuse or assault may not have life-threatening problems, but they have special needs that relate to their mental well-being. There may also be time requirements for collecting samples for evidence, and there may be local protocols for the use of assault teams and community services. Victims of acute sexual assault (within 2 hours) should be assigned level 2; others could be level 3 or less depending on the nature of the injuries or medical condition. These patients require a safe and caring environment with emotional support.

## SEVERE DRUG WITHDRAWAL

Seizures, coma, hallucinations, confusion, agitation, shakes, tremors, tachycardia, delirium tremens, hypertension, fever, chest or abdominal pain, vomiting, and diarrhea are all part of a spectrum of signs and symptoms associated with drug or alcohol withdrawal. These patients are at risk for rapid deterioration and should therefore be assigned level 2.

## CHEMOTHERAPY

Patients on chemotherapy or immunocompromised patients (e.g., HIV, known immune deficiency, malignancy), with or without a fever, are at higher risk of serious problems. These patients can deteriorate quickly and may require isolation.

# Level 3—Urgent

Level 3 represents conditions that could progress to a serious problem requiring emergency intervention. They may be associated with significant discomfort or may affect the patient's ability to function at work or in activities of daily living.

These patients have vital signs at the upper or lower limits of normal, but their presenting problem suggests a more serious acute process. They often have moderate pain (4–7/10). It is with this category of patient that the pain scales are most useful in assigning acuity.

Level 3 patients are generally stable but may have moderate pain. There is less risk of significant deterioration during transport than with higher levels of acuity. These patients can be transported to hospital without the use of lights or sirens.

**CTAS 3 guideline for time to physician in the ED is ≤30 minutes.**

The following are the usual presentations.

## HEAD INJURY

These patients may have had a head injury caused by a low-risk mechanism. (High-risk mechanisms are assigned a level 2.) They are alert (GCS 13–15) and often have a moderate headache (4–7/10) with nausea or vomiting. This includes any patient with amnesia or LOC <5 minutes.

## MODERATE TRAUMA

This category includes patients with obvious fractures or dislocations or extremity injury with severe pain (8–10/10). Dislocations should be reduced promptly, so physician assessment in the ED should occur in ≤30 minutes. Patients are stable, with normal or near-normal vital signs, often with an isolated tachycardia in response to the pain.

## MILD OR MODERATE ASTHMA

Patient may have mild to moderate SOB with exertion, frequent cough, or night awakening or may be unable to lie down flat without symptoms and have an $O_2$ saturation of 92–94%. Some documentation of medications and previous attack patterns (intubated, ICU, frequent hospital admissions) can help identify higher-risk individuals. It is unwise to assign a low triage level (4 or 5) to

an asthmatic who has called because of increased respiratory symptoms.

## MODERATE DYSPNEA

Patients with pneumonia, COPD, upper respiratory tract infection (URI), or croup may appear to be short of breath or complain of SOB. Objective assessment measures such as $O_2$ saturation are helpful, particularly if wheezing is present or the patient is known to have COPD.

## CHEST PAIN

Sharp, localized pains that become worse with deep breathing, cough, movement, or palpation and that are *not* associated with SOB or other signs that might suggest significant heart or lung disease can be assigned level 3. Vital signs should be normal.

## GASTROINTESTINAL BLEEDING

A small amount of upper or lower GI bleeding can be assigned level 3 if the patient is not actively bleeding and has normal vital signs.

## VAGINAL BLEEDING OR PELVIC PAIN

Patients with mild pelvic pain (≤4/10) and minor bleeding with normal vital signs can be assigned level 3. This includes patients in the first trimester of pregnancy with normal vital signs. Note that *any* third-trimester bleeding is level 1.

## SEIZURE

Patients with a known seizure disorder or new onset of seizure of brief duration (<5 minutes) can be assigned level 3 if they have become stable and alert, are breathing normally, are protecting their airway (normal gag), and have normal vital signs.

## ACUTE PSYCHOSIS OR SUICIDAL IMPULSES

Psychiatric problems can be assigned level 3 if the patient is not agitated and if you are uncertain whether the patient is a threat to himself or herself or to others. This applies only when there is no reason to believe that there has been a toxic ingestion and when vital signs are normal.

## SEVERE ACUTE PAIN

Patients with minor problems but self-reported intense pain (8–10/10) should have early access to physician assessment. Patients with disc-related back pain usually have a very sudden pain while lifting or bending. Radiation of pain to the legs is common. If there is muscle weakness, loss of sensation, inability to urinate, or incontinence, then more serious neurological problems may be present and urgent physician assessment is necessary (level 2).

## MODERATE ACUTE PAIN

Patients with migraine, abdominal pain, or renal colic can present with moderate pain (4–7/10). These patients would probably benefit from earlier intervention. Some moderate nontraumatic back pain can have potentially serious causes. For assignment of level 3, the patient should have normal vital signs.

## VOMITING OR DIARRHEA IN CHILDREN UNDER 2 YEARS

Dehydration and serious infections can sometimes be subtle in very young children, and vital signs may be normal. Children under 2 with vomiting and diarrhea can have significant dehydration that is not well recognized. Even if they look well, level 3 is appropriate.

# Level 4—Less Urgent

Level 4 describes conditions that are not life threatening. However, because of the patient's age, distress, or potential for deterioration or complications, the patient would benefit from intervention or reassurance within 1 hour.

These patients have stable vital signs and lower pain scales. The problem, based on the chief complaint, is not as potentially serious as in higher levels. Patients often can wait for longer times before they are seen. Patients in this category generally do not rely on an ambulance for transport to hospital.

Level 4 patients are typically very stable. These patients should be transported to hospital without lights or sirens. Many hospitals will not wish to be informed of these patients prior to arrival.

**CTAS 4 guideline for time to physician in the ED is ≤1 hour.**

The following are the usual presentations.

## HEAD INJURY

Minor scalp or head injury can be assigned level 4 if the patient has normal vital signs and is alert (GCS 15), with no LOC or amnesia, no vomiting, and no neck symptoms. The patient may have headache and nausea that are not severe.

## MINOR TRAUMA

This category includes minor fractures, sprains, contusions, abrasions, and lacerations requiring investigation or intervention. Vital signs are normal, and pain is moderate (4–7/10).

## ABDOMINAL PAIN

Acute abdominal pain of moderate intensity (4–7/10) may be assigned level 4 if vital signs are normal and if the patient does not appear to be in acute distress. Constipation can cause severe pain and on occasion can be confused with more serious problems. Start by assuming the worst possible, and ensure that there is sufficient information to exclude more urgent problems.

## HEADACHE

Headache may be assigned level 4 when it is not sudden, not severe, not migraine, and has no associated high-risk features (see level 2 and 3 headache). Infections such as sinusitis, URI, or flu-like illnesses may cause such headaches.

## EARACHE

Otitis media and externa can cause moderate (4–7/10) or severe (8–10/10) pain. Severe pain or acute distress, especially in a child, may indicate an acuity level of 3.

## CHEST PAIN

Chest pain may be assigned level 4 when the patient has normal vital signs, no acute distress, no more than moderate pain (4–7/10), no SOB, no visceral features, and no previous heart problems. These patients may have had a chest wall injury or some strain of the muscles from cough or physical activity.

## SUICIDAL FEELINGS OR DEPRESSION

Patients complaining of passive suicidal thoughts (that is, with no impulse to act on them) and who do not seem agitated may be assigned level 4.

## CORNEAL FOREIGN BODY

Level 4 is appropriate if pain is mild or moderate (4–7/10) and there is no change in visual acuity.

## CHRONIC BACK PAIN

These patients may be very challenging and should always be assessed as though their problem has never been seen before. It is usually easy to confirm that the pattern is identical to earlier pain and that neurological abnormalities are not present.

## UPPER RESPIRATORY INFECTION SYMPTOMS

Patients with upper airway congestion, cough, aches, fever, and sore throat are frequent visitors to the ED. If there are significant respiratory signs or symptoms or if $O_2$ saturation is <95%, upgrade the acuity level.

## VOMITING AND/OR DIARRHEA WITH NO SIGNS OF DEHYDRATION (AGE >2)

The risk of dehydration increases with vomiting and diarrhea together. Questions should attempt to clearly define the onset and course of the illness with quantification of the episodes of diarrhea and vomiting. If there are fewer than five loose bowel movements per day, then dehydration or electrolyte imbalances are unlikely.

## MODERATE ACUTE PAIN

Moderate pain (4–7/10) with minor injuries or musculoskeletal problems may be assigned level 4.

# Level 5—Nonurgent

This level includes acute but nonurgent conditions, as well as conditions that may be part of a chronic problem, with or without evidence of deterioration. These patients often do not call the ambulance but find their own way to a hospital. These are truly minor complaints that do not pose any immediate risk to the patient.

Level 5 patients are stable and are transported on a routine basis.

**CTAS 5 guideline for time to physician in the ED is ≤2 hours.**

The following are the usual presentations.

## MINOR TRAUMA

Injuries in this category include contusions, abrasions, minor lacerations not requiring closure by any means, overuse syndromes (e.g., tendonitis), and sprains.

## SORE THROAT, UPPER RESPIRATORY INFECTIONS

This category includes patients with minor complaints characteristic of typical viral illnesses and with no respiratory symptoms or compromise. Vital signs are normal, or there may be a low-grade fever.

## VAGINAL BLEEDING

Bleeding may be a normal period or painless bleeding in postmenopausal patients. Patients have normal vital signs.

## ABDOMINAL PAIN

Patients in this category have normal vital signs and mild pain (<4/10) that is chronic or recurring.

## VOMITING ALONE OR DIARRHEA ALONE, WITH NO SIGNS OF DEHYDRATION AND AGE >2

These patients should have normal mental status and vital signs.

## PSYCHIATRIC

These patients may seem to have minor or insignificant problems from the healthcare provider's point of view but may be frustrated by the lack of other healthcare options in the community. They may also simply be unaware of what other options are available. Having an open mind and being sensitive to socioeconomic and cultural issues will allow you to evaluate the level of care needed and the risk of harm to self or others.

## Patients for Whom It Is Hard to Assign an Acuity Level

Sometimes it is difficult to assign an acuity level because the patient does not seem to fit any of the categories. In this case, you need to either discuss the case with your partner or make a judgment based on experience or instinct. The fundamental consideration is the potential seriousness of the problem and how quickly it needs to be dealt with. When in doubt, always err on the side of assigning a higher level of acuity. See Figure B–1 on the next page for a summary of levels and usual presentations.

## REFERENCES

Beveridge RC. The Canadian Triage and Acuity Scale: A new and critical element in health care reform. *J Emerg Med.* 1998; 16:507–511.

Beveridge RC, Clarke B, Janes L, Savage N, Thompson J, Dodd G, Murray M, Nijssen-Jordan C, Warren D, Vadeboncoeur A: Canadian Emergency Department Triage and Acuity Scale: Implementation Guidelines. *Can J Emerg Med.* 1999; 1(3) (Suppl).

Beveridge RC, Ducharme J, Janes L, Beaulieu S, Walter S. Reliability of the Canadian Emergency Department Triage and Acuity interrater agreement. *Ann Emerg Med.* 1999;34:155–159.

Jelinek G, Little M. Interrater reliability of the National Triage Scale. *Emerg Med.* 1996; 8:226–230.

Australasian College of Emergency Medicine. National Triage Scale. Policy document. *Emerg Med.* 1994;6:145–146.

Erwich-Nijhout M, Bond M, Baggoley C. *Report to the Commonwealth Department of Health and Family Services: Costings in the Emergency Department.* 1996.

Warren D, Jarvis A, LeBlanc L, Beveridge R, Murray M, Thompson J, Dodd G, Nijssen- Jordan C, Vadeboncoeur A, O'Brien J, Belanger F: Pediatric Canadian Emergency Department Triage and Acuity Scale. *Can J Emerg Med.* 2001.

The Canadian Association of Emergency Physicians
L'Association canadienne des médecins d'urgence

NENA National Emergency Nurses Affiliation Inc.
L'affiliation nationale des infirmières/infirmiers d'urgence incorporée

L'ASSOCIATION DES MÉDECINS D'URGENCE DU QUÉBEC

# The Canadian E.D. Triage and Acuity Scale

Patients should have an
**INITIAL TRIAGE ASSESSMENT WITHIN 10 MINUTES** of arrival

## TRIAGE LEVEL I - RESUSCITATION

Time to NURSE Assessment **IMMEDIATE***
Time to PHYSICIAN Assessment **IMMEDIATE***

| USUAL PRESENTATION | SENTINEL DIAGNOSIS |
|---|---|
| Code / Arrest | Traumatic Shock |
| Major Trauma | Pneumothorax - Traumatic / Tension |
| Shock States | Facial Burns with Airway Compromise |
| Near Death Asthma | Severe Burns > 30% TBS |
| Severe Respiratory Distress | Overdose with Hypotension / Unconscious |
| Altered Mental State (unconscious, delerious) | AAA |
| Seizures | AMI with Complications / CHF / Low BP |
| | Status Asthmaticus |
| | Head Injury - Major / Unconscious |
| | Status Epilepticus |

## TRIAGE LEVEL II - EMERGENT

Time to NURSE Assessment **IMMEDIATE***
Time to PHYSICIAN Assessment **15 MINUTES***

| USUAL PRESENTATION | SENTINEL DIAGNOSIS |
|---|---|
| Head Injury (Risk Features ± Altered Mental State) | Head Injury |
| Severe Trauma | Trauma, Multiple Sites, Multiple Rib Fracture, Neck Injury / Spinal Cord |
| Altered Mental State (lethargic, drowsy, agitated) | |
| Chemical Exposure - Eyes | Alkaline / Caustic Ocular Burns |
| Allergic Reaction (Severe) | Anaphylaxis |
| Chest Pain • Visceral, Non-Traumatic | AMI, Unstable Angina, CHF, Chest Pain NOS, |
| • ± Associated Symptoms | Gastroesophageal Reflux |
| Overdose (conscious), Drug Withdrawal | Unspecified Drug / Medicinal Overdose, "d.t.'s" |
| ABD Pain (Age >50) with Visceral Symptoms | AAA, Appendicitis, Cholecystitis |
| Back Pain (Non Trauma, Not MSK) | |
| GI Bleed with Abnormal Vital Signs | Gastrointestinal Bleed, Hypotension |
| CVA with Major Deficit | CVA |
| Asthma Severe (PEFR <40%) | Severe Asthma |
| Moderate / Severe Dyspnea / Difficulty Breathing | COPD, Croup |
| Vaginal Bleeding • Acute, Pain scale >5 | Spontaneous Abortion |
| • ± Abnormal Vital Signs | Ectopic Pregnancy / Rupture |
| Vomiting and/or diarrhea (with suspicion of dehydration) | |
| Signs of serious infection (purpuric rash, toxic) | |
| Chemotherapy or immunocompromised | |
| Fever (age ≤3 months) Temp ≥ 38.0 (rectal) | Epiglottitis, Meningitis, Sepsis |
| Acute Psychotic Episode / Extreme Agitation | Acute Psychotic Episode / Agitation |
| Diabetes: Hypoglycemia, Hyperglycemia | Hypoglycemia, Diabetic Ketoacidosis, Hyperglycemia |
| Headache (Pain Scale 8 - 10/10) | Migraine |
| Pain Scale 8-10 (CVA, Back, Eye) | Renal Colic, LBP / Strain (Disc), Keratitis, Iritis |
| Sexual Assault | |
| Neonate (≤7 days old) | |

## TRIAGE LEVEL III - URGENT

Time to NURSE Assessment **30 MINUTES***
Time to PHYSICIAN Assessment **30 MINUTES***

| USUAL PRESENTATION | SENTINEL DIAGNOSIS |
|---|---|
| Head Injury, Alert, Vomiting | Head Injury |
| Moderate Trauma | Dislocated Shoulder, Tibia / Fibula Fracture, Bimalleolar, Trimalleolar Ankle Fracture |
| Abuse / Neglect / Assault | |
| Vomiting and/or diarrhea (≤2 years) | |
| Dialysis problems | |
| Signs of Infection | Pyelonephritis |
| Mild / Moderate Asthma (PEFR > 40%) | Asthma without Status |
| Mild / Moderate Dyspnea | Bronchiolitis / Croup, Pneumonia, COPD |
| Chest Pain • No Visceral Symptoms (Sharp/MSK) | Chest Pain NOS (MSK, GI, Resp) |
| • No Previous Heart Disease | |
| GI Bleed with Normal Vital Signs | GI Bleed, No complications |
| Vaginal Bleeding Acute, Normal Vital Signs | Spontaneous Abortion |
| Seizure, Alert on Arrival | Seizure |
| Acute Psychosis ± Suicidal Ideation | Acute Psychosis ± Suicidal Ideation |
| Pain Scale 8 - 10 / 10 with minor injuries | |
| Pain Scale 4 - 7 / 10 (Headache, CVA, Back) | Migraine, Renal Colic, LBP / Strain (Disc) |

## TRIAGE LEVEL IV - LESS URGENT

Time to NURSE Assessment **60 MINUTES***
Time to PHYSICIAN Assessment **60 MINUTES***

| USUAL PRESENTATION | SENTINEL DIAGNOSIS |
|---|---|
| Head Injury, Alert, No Vomiting | Head Injury, Alert, No Vomiting |
| Minor Trauma | Colles Fracture, Ankle Sprain |
| ABD Pain (Acute) | Appendicitis, Cholecystitis |
| Earache | Otitis Media / Otitis Externa |
| Chest Pain, Minor Trauma or MSK, No Distress | Chest Pain NOS (MSK, GI, Resp), Gastroesophageal Reflux |
| Vomiting and diarrhea (>2 years/no dehydration) | |
| Suicidal Ideation / Depression | Suicidal Ideation / Depression |
| Allergic Reaction (Minor) | Urticaria |
| Corneal Foreign Body | Corneal Foreign Body |
| Back Pain (Chronic) | LBP / Strain |
| URI Symptoms | URI |
| Pain Scale 4 - 7 | |
| Headache (Non Migraine / Not Sudden) | |

## TRIAGE LEVEL V - NON URGENT

Time to NURSE Assessment **120 MINUTES***
Time to PHYSICIAN Assessment **120 MINUTES***

| USUAL PRESENTATION | SENTINEL DIAGNOSIS |
|---|---|
| Minor Trauma, Not Necessarily Acute | LBP / Strain |
| Sore Throat, No Resp Symptoms | URI |
| Diarrhea alone (no dehydration) | Gastroenteritis |
| Vomiting alone normal mental status (no dehydration) | Vomiting |
| Menses | Disorders of Menstruation |
| Minor Symptoms | Dressing Changes |
| ABD Pain (Chronic) | Cast Changes |
| Psychiatric complaints | Constipation |
| Pain Scale < 4 | Symptoms / Neurotic, Personality and Nonpsychotic Mental Disorders |
| | Unspecified Superficial Laceration(s) |

*****TIMES TO ASSESSMENT** are operating objectives, not established standards of care. Facilities without onsite physician coverage may meet assessment objectives using delegated protocols and remote communication.

**FIGURE B-1** The Canadian triage and acuity scale.

# APPENDIX C
# National Occupational Competency Profiles (NOCP)

## PRIMARY CARE PARAMEDIC AND ADVANCED CARE PARAMEDIC COMPETENCIES

The following table indicates the level or educational stage or environment in which the paramedic is expected to achieve the competencies. The reference chapters reflect the theory for the competencies.

**N** The competency is *not applicable* to the practitioner.

**X** The practitioner should have a *basic awareness* of the subject matter of the competency.

**A** The practitioner must have demonstrated an *academic understanding* of the competency.

**S** The practitioner must have demonstrated the competency in a simulated setting. Individual evaluation of physical application skills is required, utilizing any of the following: practical scenario, skill station, mannequin, cadaver, live subject (human or nonhuman). In Competency Areas 4 and 5, skills must be demonstrated on a human subject, where legally and ethically acceptable.

**C** The practitioner must have demonstrated the competency in a clinical setting with a patient.

**P** The practitioner must have demonstrated the competency in a field preceptorship with a patient.

MPT = *Mosby's Paramedic Textbook*
TCP = *The Canadian Paramedic: An Introduction*

## SPECIFIC COMPETENCY

## Area 1 Professional Responsibilities

### GENERAL COMPETENCY 1.1 FUNCTION AS A PROFESSIONAL.

| | | PCP | ACP | Reference: Chapters |
|---|---|---|---|---|
| 1.1.a | Maintain patient dignity. | P | P | MPT: 2, 5, 10, 40 |
| 1.1.b | Reflect professionalism through use of appropriate language. | P | P | MPT: 1, 9, 15 |
| 1.1.c | Dress appropriately, and maintain personal hygiene. | P | P | MPT:1, 2 |
| 1.1.d | Maintain appropriate personal interaction with patients. | A | A | MPT: 9 |
| 1.1.e | Maintain patient confidentiality. | P | P | MPT: 1, 4, 5 |
| 1.1.f | Participate in quality assurance and enhancement programs. | A | A | MPT: 1 TCP: 1 |
| 1.1.g | Utilize community support agencies as appropriate. | A | A | MPT: 1 |
| 1.1.h | Promote awareness of emergency medical system and profession. | P | P | MPT: 1 |
| 1.1.i | Participate in a professional association. | A | A | MPT: 1 TCP: 1 |
| 1.1.j | Behave ethically. | P | P | MPT: 5 TCP: 1, 3 |
| 1.1.k | Function as patient advocate. | P | P | MPT: 1, 5 TCP: 1, 2 |

## GENERAL COMPETENCY 1.2
## PARTICIPATE IN CONTINUING EDUCATION.

| | | | |
|---|---|---|---|
| 1.2.a | Develop personal plan for continuing professional development. | A    A | MPT: 1 TCP: 1 |
| 1.2.b | Self-evaluate, and set goals for improvement, as related to professional practice. | A    A | MPT: 1 TCP: 1 |
| 1.2.c | Interpret evidence in medical literature, and assess relevance to practice. | A    A | MPT: 1 |

## GENERAL COMPETENCY 1.3
## POSSESS AN UNDERSTANDING OF THE
## MEDICO-LEGAL ASPECTS OF THE PROFESSION.

| | | | |
|---|---|---|---|
| 1.3.a | Comply with scope of practice. | P    P | MPT: 4 TCP: 1 |
| 1.3.b | Recognize "patient rights" and the implications on the role of the provider. | A    A | MPT: 4, 5 TCP:1, 3 |
| 1.3.c | Include all pertinent and required information on ambulance call report forms. | P    P | MPT: 16 TCP: 1,3 |

## GENERAL COMPETENCY 1.4
## RECOGNIZE AND COMPLY WITH
## RELEVANT PROVINCIAL AND FEDERAL LEGISLATION.

| | | | |
|---|---|---|---|
| 1.4.a | Function within relevant legislation, policies, and procedures. | A    A | MPT: 4, TCP: 3 |

## GENERAL COMPETENCY 1.5
## FUNCTION EFFECTIVELY IN A TEAM ENVIRONMENT.

| | | | |
|---|---|---|---|
| 1.5.a | Work collaboratively with a partner. | P    P | MPT: 14 TCP: 1 |
| 1.5.b | Accept and deliver constructive feedback. | P    P | MPT: 1 TCP: 1 |
| 1.5.c | Work collaboratively with other emergency response agencies. | P    P | MPT: 1 TCP: 1 |
| 1.5.d | Work collaboratively with other members of the healthcare team. | P    P | MPT: 1 TCP: 1 |

## GENERAL COMPETENCY 1.6
## MAKE DECISIONS EFFECTIVELY.

| | | | |
|---|---|---|---|
| 1.6.a | Exhibit reasonable and prudent judgment. | P    P | MPT: 1, 5, 13 TCP: 3 |
| 1.6.b | Practise effective problem-solving. | P    P | MPT: 13, 14 |
| 1.6.c | Delegate tasks appropriately. | P    P | MPT: 13, 14 |

# Area 2 Communication

## GENERAL COMPETENCY 2.1
## PRACTISE EFFECTIVE ORAL COMMUNICATION SKILLS.

| | | PCP | ACP | Reference: Chapters |
|---|---|---|---|---|
| 2.1.a | Deliver an organized, accurate, and relevant report utilizing telecommunication devices. | P | P | MPT: 15 |
| 2.1.b | Deliver an organized, accurate, and relevant verbal report. | P | P | MPT: 15 |
| 2.1.c | Deliver an organized, accurate, and relevant patient history. | P | P | MPT: 10 |
| 2.1.d | Provide information to patients about their situation and how they will be treated. | P | P | MPT: 4, 9 |
| 2.1.e | Interact effectively with the patient, relatives, and bystanders who are in stressful situations. | P | P | MPT: 9 |
| 2.1.f | Speak in language appropriate to the listener. | P | P | MPT: 8, 9 |
| 2.1.g | Use appropriate terminology. | P | P | MPT: 15 |

## GENERAL COMPETENCY 2.2
## PRACTISE EFFECTIVE WRITTEN COMMUNICATION SKILLS.

| | | | | |
|---|---|---|---|---|
| 2.2.a | Record organized, accurate, and relevant patient information. | P | P | MPT: 16 |
| 2.2.b | Prepare professional correspondence. | A | A | MPT: 16 |

## GENERAL COMPETENCY 2.3
## PRACTISE EFFECTIVE NONVERBAL COMMUNICATION SKILLS.

| | | | |
|---|---|---|---|
| 2.3.a Exhibit effective nonverbal behaviour. | S | S | MPT: 9 |
| 2.3.b Practise active listening techniques. | P | P | MPT: 9 |
| 2.3.c Establish trust and rapport with patients and colleagues. | P | P | MPT: 9 TCP: 1 |
| 2.3.d Recognize and react appropriately to nonverbal behaviours. | P | P | MPT: 9 |

## GENERAL COMPETENCY 2.4
## PRACTISE EFFECTIVE INTERPERSONAL RELATIONS.

| | | | |
|---|---|---|---|
| 2.4.a Treat others with respect. | P | P | MPT: 9 |
| 2.4.b Exhibit empathy and compassion while providing care. | P | P | MPT: 9 TCP: 1 |
| 2.4.c Recognize and react appropriately to individuals and groups manifesting coping mechanisms. | P | P | MPT: 9, 40 |
| 2.4.d Act in a confident manner. | P | P | MPT: 9 |
| 2.4.e Act assertively as required. | P | P | MPT: 9 |
| 2.4.f Manage and provide support to patients, bystanders, and relatives manifesting emotional reactions. | P | P | MPT: 9 |
| 2.4.g Exhibit diplomacy, tact, and discretion. | P | P | MPT: 9 TCP: 1 |
| 2.4.h Exhibit conflict resolution skills. | S | S | MPT: 9 TCP: 1 |

# Area 3 Health and Safety

## GENERAL COMPETENCY 3.1
## MAINTAIN GOOD PHYSICAL AND MENTAL HEALTH.

| | PCP | ACP | Reference: Chapters |
|---|---|---|---|
| 3.1.a Maintain balance in personal lifestyle. | A | A | MPT: 2 |
| 3.1.b Develop and maintain an appropriate support system. | A | A | MPT: 2 |
| 3.1.c Manage personal stress. | A | A | MPT: 2 |
| 3.1.d Practise effective strategies to improve physical and mental health related to shift work. | A | A | MPT: 2 |
| 3.1.e Exhibit physical strength and fitness consistent with the requirements of professional practice. | P | P | MPT: 2 |

## GENERAL COMPETENCY 3.2
## PRACTISE SAFE LIFTING AND MOVING TECHNIQUES.

| | | | |
|---|---|---|---|
| 3.2.a Practise safe biomechanics. | P | P | MPT: 2 |
| 3.2.b Transfer patient from various positions using applicable equipment and/or techniques. | P | P | MPT: 1, 49 |
| 3.2.c Transfer patient using emergency evacuation techniques. | S | S | MPT: 49, 51 |
| 3.2.d Secure patient to applicable equipment. | P | P | MPT: 51 |
| 3.2.e Lift patient and stretcher in and out of ambulance with partner. | P | P | MPT: 2 |

## GENERAL COMPETENCY 3.3
## CREATE AND MAINTAIN A SAFE WORK ENVIRONMENT.

| | | | |
|---|---|---|---|
| 3.3.a Assess scene for safety. | P | P | MPT: 1, 2 |
| 3.3.b Address potential occupational hazards. | P | P | MPT: 2, 53, 54 |
| 3.3.c Conduct basic extrication. | S | S | MPT: 50 |
| 3.3.d Exhibit defusing and self-protection behaviours appropriate for use with patients and bystanders. | S | S | MPT: 40 |
| 3.3.e Conduct procedures and operations consistent with Workplace Hazardous Materials Information System (WHMIS) and hazardous materials management requirements. | A | A | MPT: 53 |
| 3.3.f Practise infection control techniques. | P | P | MPT: 2, 39 |
| 3.3.g Clean and disinfect equipment. | P | P | MPT: 39 |
| 3.3.h Clean and disinfect an emergency vehicle. | P | P | MPT: 39 |

# Area 4 Assessment and Diagnosis

## GENERAL COMPETENCY 4.1 CONDUCT TRIAGE.

| | | PCP | ACP | Reference: Chapters |
|---|---|---|---|---|
| 4.1.a | Rapidly assess a scene based on the principles of a triage system. | S | S | MPT: 50 |
| 4.1.b | Assume different roles in a mass casualty incident. | A | A | MPT: 50 |
| 4.1.c | Manage a mass casualty incident. | A | A | MPT: 50 |

## GENERAL COMPETENCY 4.2 OBTAIN PATIENT HISTORY.

| | | PCP | ACP | |
|---|---|---|---|---|
| 4.2.a | Obtain list of patient's allergies. | P | P | MPT: 10 |
| 4.2.b | Obtain list of patient's medications. | P | P | MPT: 10 |
| 4.2.c | Obtain chief complaint and/or incident history from patient, family members, and/or bystanders. | P | P | MPT: 10, 12 |
| 4.2.d | Obtain information regarding patient's past medical history. | P | P | MPT: 10 |
| 4.2.e | Obtain information about patient's last oral intake. | P | P | MPT: 10 |
| 4.2.f | Obtain information regarding incident through accurate and complete scene assessment. | P | P | MPT: 12 |

## GENERAL COMPETENCY 4.3
## CONDUCT COMPLETE PHYSICAL ASSESSMENT DEMONSTRATING APPROPRIATE USE OF INSPECTION, PALPATION, PERCUSSION, AND AUSCULTATION, AND INTERPRET FINDINGS.

| | | PCP | ACP | |
|---|---|---|---|---|
| 4.3.a | Conduct primary patient assessment, and interpret findings. | P | P | MPT: 11, 12 |
| 4.3.b | Conduct secondary patient assessment, and interpret findings. | P | P | MPT: 11, 12 |
| 4.3.c | Conduct cardiovascular system assessment, and interpret findings. | P | P | MPT: 11, 12, 29 |
| 4.3.d | Conduct neurological system assessment, and interpret findings. | P | P | MPT: 11, 12, 31 |
| 4.3.e | Conduct respiratory system assessment, and interpret findings. | P | P | MPT: 11, 12, 30 |
| 4.3.f | Conduct obstetrical assessment, and interpret findings. | S | C | MPT: 11, 12, 42 |
| 4.3.g | Conduct gastrointestinal system assessment, and interpret findings. | S | P | MPT: 11, 12, 34 |
| 4.3.h | Conduct genitourinary system assessment, and interpret findings. | S | P | MPT: 11, 12, 35 |
| 4.3.i | Conduct integumentary system assessment, and interpret findings. | S | S | MPT: 11, 12, 22, 39 |
| 4.3.j | Conduct musculoskeletal assessment, and interpret findings. | P | P | MPT: 11, 12, 28 |
| 4.3.k | Conduct assessment of the immune system, and interpret findings. | P | P | MPT: 33 |
| 4.3.l | Conduct assessment of the endocrine system, and interpret findings. | P | P | MPT: 32 |
| 4.3.m | Conduct assessment of the ears, eyes, nose and throat, and interpret findings. | S | S | MPT: 11, 12 |
| 4.3.n | Conduct multisystem assessment, and interpret findings. | P | P | MPT: 11, 12 |
| 4.3.o | Conduct neonatal assessment, and interpret findings. | S | C | MPT: 43 |
| 4.3.p | Conduct psychiatric assessment, and interpret findings. | S | S | MPT: 40 |

## GENERAL COMPETENCY 4.4 ASSESS VITAL SIGNS.

| | | PCP | ACP | |
|---|---|---|---|---|
| 4.4.a | Assess pulse. | P | P | MPT: 11, 12 |
| 4.4.b | Assess respiration. | P | P | MPT: 11, 12 |
| 4.4.c | Conduct noninvasive temperature monitoring. | C | C | MPT: 11, 12 |
| 4.4.d | Measure blood pressure by auscultation. | P | P | MPT: 11, 12 |
| 4.4.e | Measure blood pressure by palpation. | P | P | MPT: 11, 12 |
| 4.4.f | Measure blood pressure with noninvasive blood pressure monitor. | C | C | MPT: 11, 12 |
| 4.4.g | Assess skin condition. | P | P | MPT: 11, 12 |
| 4.4.h | Assess pupils. | P | P | MPT: 11, 12 |
| 4.4.i | Assess level of mentation. | P | P | MPT: 11, 12 |

## GENERAL COMPETENCY 4.5 UTILIZE DIAGNOSTIC TESTS.

| | | PCP | ACP | |
|---|---|---|---|---|
| 4.5.a | Conduct oximetry testing, and interpret findings. | C | C | MPT: 19, 30 |
| 4.5.b | Conduct end-tidal carbon dioxide monitoring and interpret findings. | N | C | MPT: 11, 19, 30 |

| | PCP | ACP | Reference: Chapters |
|---|---|---|---|
| 4.5.c Conduct glucometric testing, and interpret findings. | P | P | MPT: 32 |
| 4.5.d Conduct peripheral venipuncture. | N | X | MPT: 18 |
| 4.5.e Obtain arterial blood samples via radial artery puncture. | N | X | MPT: 18, 19, Appendix |
| 4.5.f Obtain arterial blood samples via arterial line access. | N | X | MPT: 19, Appendix |
| 4.5.g Conduct invasive core temperature monitoring, and interpret findings. | N | X | MPT: 11, Appendix |
| 4.5.h Conduct pulmonary artery catheter monitoring, and interpret findings. | N | X | MPT: 19, Appendix |
| 4.5.i Conduct central venous pressure monitoring, and interpret findings. | N | X | MPT: 19, Appendix |
| 4.5.j Conduct arterial line monitoring, and interpret findings. | N | X | MPT: 18, 19, Appendix |
| 4.5.k Interpret laboratory and radiological data. | X | A | MPT: Appendix |
| 4.5.l Conduct 3-lead electrocardiogram (ECG), and interpret findings. | S | P | MPT: 29 |
| 4.5.m Obtain 12-lead electrocardiogram, and interpret findings. | X | A | MPT: 29 |

# Area 5 Therapeutics

### GENERAL COMPETENCY 5.1
### MAINTAIN PATENCY OF UPPER AIRWAY AND TRACHEA.

| | PCP | ACP | Reference: Chapters |
|---|---|---|---|
| 5.1.a Use manual manoeuvres and positioning to maintain airway patency. | C | C | MPT: 19 |
| 5.1.b Suction oropharynx. | S | C | MPT: 19 |
| 5.1.c Suction beyond oropharynx. | A | C | MPT: 19 |
| 5.1 d Utilize oropharyngeal airway. | S | C | MPT: 19 |
| 5.1.e Utilize nasopharyngeal airway. | S | S | MPT: 19 |
| 5.1.f Utilize airway devices not requiring visualization of vocal cords and not introduced endotracheally. | A | S | MPT: 19 |
| 5.1.g Utilize airway devices not requiring visualization of vocal cords and introduced endotracheally. | A | S | MPT: 19 |
| 5.1.h Utilize airway devices requiring visualization of vocal cords and introduced endotracheally. | A | C | MPT: 19 |
| 5.1.i Remove airway foreign bodies (AFB). | S | S | MPT: 19 |
| 5.1.j Remove foreign body by direct techniques. | X | S | MPT: 19 |
| 5.1.k Conduct percutaneous cricothyroidotomy. | X | S | MPT: 19 |
| 5.1.l Conduct surgical cricothyroidotomy. | N | A | MPT: 19 |

### GENERAL COMPETENCY 5.2 PREPARE OXYGEN DELIVERY DEVICES.

| | PCP | ACP | Reference: Chapters |
|---|---|---|---|
| 5.2.a Recognize indications for oxygen administration. | A | A | MPT: 19 |
| 5.2.b Take appropriate safety precautions. | A | A | MPT: 19 |
| 5.2.c Ensure adequacy of oxygen supply. | A | A | MPT: 19 |
| 5.2.d Recognize different types of oxygen delivery systems. | A | A | MPT: 19 |
| 5.2.e Utilize portable oxygen delivery systems. | P | P | MPT: 19 |

### GENERAL COMPETENCY 5.3
### DELIVER OXYGEN, AND ADMINISTER MANUAL VENTILATION.

| | PCP | ACP | Reference: Chapters |
|---|---|---|---|
| 5.3.a Administer oxygen using nasal cannula. | C | C | MPT: 19 |
| 5.3.b Administer oxygen using low-concentration mask. | C | C | MPT: 19 |
| 5.3.c Administer oxygen using controlled-concentration mask. | X | X | MPT: 19 |
| 5.3.d Administer oxygen using high-concentration mask. | C | C | MPT: 19 |
| 5.3.e Administer oxygen using pocket mask. | S | S | MPT: 19 |

### GENERAL COMPETENCY 5.4 UTILIZE VENTILATION EQUIPMENT.

| | PCP | ACP | Reference: Chapters |
|---|---|---|---|
| 5.4.a Provide oxygenation and ventilation using bag-valve-mask. | C | C | MPT: 19 |
| 5.4.b Recognize indications for mechanical ventilation. | A | A | MPT: 19 |
| 5.4.c Prepare mechanical ventilation equipment. | A | A | MPT: 19 |
| 5.4.d Provide mechanical ventilation. | N | C | MPT: 19 |

## GENERAL COMPETENCY 5.5
## IMPLEMENT MEASURES TO MAINTAIN HEMODYNAMIC STABILITY.

| | | | |
|---|---|---|---|
| 5.5.a Conduct cardiopulmonary resuscitation (CPR). | S | S | MPT: 29 |
| 5.5.b Control external hemorrhage through the use of direct pressure and patient positioning. | S | S | MPT: 21 |
| 5.5 c Maintain peripheral intravenous (IV) access devices and infusions of crystalloid solutions without additives. | C | P | MPT: 18 |
| 5.5.d Conduct peripheral intravenous cannulation. | A | P | MPT: 18 |
| 5.5.e Conduct intraosseous needle insertion. | X | S | MPT: 18 |
| 5.5.f Utilize direct pressure infusion devices with intravenous infusions. | A | S | MPT: 18 |
| 5.5.g Administer volume expanders (colloid and noncrystalloid). | X | S | MPT: 18 |
| 5.5 h Administer blood and/or blood products. | X | A | MPT: Appendix |
| 5.5.i Conduct automated external defibrillation. | S | S | MPT: 29 |
| 5.5.j Conduct manual defibrillation. | X | S | MPT: 29 |
| 5.5.k Conduct cardioversion. | X | S | MPT: 29 |
| 5.5.l Conduct transcutaneous pacing. | X | S | MPT: 29 |
| 5.5.m Maintain transvenous pacing. | N | A | MPT: 29 |
| 5.5.n Maintain intra-aortic balloon pumps. | N | X | MPT: Appendix |
| 5.5.o Provide routine care for patient with urinary catheter. | S | C | MPT: 35 |
| 5.5.p Provide routine care for patient with ostomy drainage system. | A | S | MPT: 48 |
| 5.5.q Provide routine care for patient with noncatheter urinary drainage system. | A | A | MPT: 35 |
| 5.5.r Monitor chest tubes. | X | X | MPT: Appendix |
| 5.5.s Conduct needle thoracostomy. | X | S | MPT: 26 |
| 5.5.t Conduct oral and nasal gastric tube insertion. | X | S | MPT: 19 |
| 5.5.u Conduct urinary catheterization. | X | A | MPT: 53 |

## GENERAL COMPETENCY 5.6
## PROVIDE BASIC CARE FOR SOFT-TISSUE INJURIES.

| | | | |
|---|---|---|---|
| 5.6.a Treat soft-tissue injuries. | P | P | MPT: 20 |
| 5.6.b Treat burn. | S | S | MPT: 23 |
| 5.6.c Treat eye injury. | S | S | MPT: 20 |
| 5.6.d Treat penetration wound. | S | S | MPT: 20 |
| 5.6.e Treat local cold injury. | S | S | MPT: 38 |

## GENERAL COMPETENCY 5.7
## IMMOBILIZE ACTUAL AND SUSPECTED FRACTURES.

| | | | |
|---|---|---|---|
| 5.7.a Immobilize suspected fractures involving appendicular skeleton. | S | S | MPT: 28 |
| 5.7.b Immobilize suspected fractures involving axial skeleton. | P | P | MPT: 28 |

## GENERAL COMPETENCY 5.8 ADMINISTER MEDICATIONS.

| | | | |
|---|---|---|---|
| 5.8.a Recognize principles of pharmacology as applied to the medications listed in Appendix 5. | A | A | MPT: 17 TCP: Appendix A |
| 5.8.b Follow safe process for responsible medication administration. | S | P | MPT: 17 TCP: Appendix A |
| 5.8.c Administer medication via subcutaneous route. | S | C | MPT: 17 |
| 5.8.d Administer medication via intramuscular route. | S | C | MPT: 17 |
| 5.8.e Administer medication via intravenous route. | X | P | MPT: 17 |
| 5.8.f Administer medication via intraosseous route. | X | S | MPT: 17 |
| 5.8.g Administer medication via endotracheal route. | X | S | MPT: 17 |
| 5.8.h Administer medication via sublingual route. | S | C | MPT: 17 |
| 5.8.i Administer medication via topical route. | X | S | MPT: 17 |
| 5.8.j Administer medication via oral route. | S | C | MPT: 17 |
| 5.8.k Administer medication via rectal route. | X | A | MPT: 17 |
| 5.8.l Administer medication via inhalation. | S | C | MPT: 17 |

# Area 6 Integration

### GENERAL COMPETENCY 6.1
### UTILIZE DIFFERENTIAL DIAGNOSIS SKILLS,
### DECISION-MAKING SKILLS AND PSYCHOMOTOR SKILLS
### IN PROVIDING CARE TO PATIENTS.

|  |  | PCP | ACP | Reference: Chapters |
|---|---|---|---|---|
| 6.1.a | Provide care to patient experiencing illness or injury primarily involving cardiovascular system. | P | P | MPT: 26, 29 |
| 6.1.b | Provide care to patient experiencing illness or injury primarily involving neurological system. | P | P | MPT: 31 |
| 6.1.c | Provide care to patient experiencing illness or injury primarily involving respiratory system. | P | P | MPT: 19, 30 |
| 6.1.d | Provide care to patient experiencing illness or injury primarily involving genitourinary/reproductive system. | S | S | MPT: 35, 41 |
| 6.1.e | Provide care to patient experiencing illness or injury primarily involving gastrointestinal system. | P | P | MPT: 34 |
| 6.1.f | Provide care to patient experiencing illness or injury primarily involving integumentary system. | P | P | MPT: 22, 39 |
| 6.1.g | Provide care to patient experiencing illness or injury primarily involving musculoskeletal system. | P | P | MPT: 28 |
| 6.1.h | Provide care to patient experiencing illness primarily involving immune system. | S | S | MPT: 33 |
| 6.1.i | Provide care to patient experiencing illness primarily involving endocrine system. | S | S | MPT: 32 |
| 6.1.j | Provide care to patient experiencing illness or injury primarily involving the eyes, ears, nose, or throat. | S | S | MPT: 22, 24 |
| 6.1.k | Provide care to patient experiencing illness or injury due to poisoning or overdose. | S | P | MPT: 36 |
| 6.1.l | Provide care to patient experiencing nonurgent medical problem. | P | P | MPT: 48 |
| 6.1.m | Provide care to patient experiencing terminal illness. | S | S | MPT: 47, 48 |
| 6.1.n | Provide care to patient experiencing illness or injury due to extremes of temperature or adverse environments. | S | S | MPT: 38 |
| 6.1.o | Provide care to patient based on understanding of common physiological, anatomical, incident and patient-specific field trauma criteria that determine appropriate decisions for triage, transport, and destination. | P | P | MPT: 20, 50 |
| 6.1.p | Provide care for patient experiencing psychiatric crisis. | S | P | MPT: 40, 47 |
| 6.1.q | Provide care for patient in labour. | S | C | MPT: 42 |

### GENERAL COMPETENCY 6.2.
### PROVIDE CARE TO MEET THE NEEDS
### OF UNIQUE PATIENT GROUPS.

|  |  | PCP | ACP | Reference: Chapters |
|---|---|---|---|---|
| 6.2.a | Provide care for neonatal patient. | S | C | MPT: 43 |
| 6.2.b | Provide care for pediatric patient. | C | C | MPT: 44 |
| 6.2.c | Provide care for geriatric patient. | C | C | MPT: 45 |
| 6.2.d | Provide care for physically challenged patient. | S | S | MPT: 47 |
| 6.2.e | Provide care for mentally challenged patient. | S | S | MPT: 47 |

### GENERAL COMPETENCY 6.3
### CONDUCT ONGOING ASSESSMENTS, AND PROVIDE CARE.

|  |  | PCP | ACP | Reference: Chapters |
|---|---|---|---|---|
| 6.3.a | Conduct ongoing assessments based on patient presentation, and interpret findings. | P | P | MPT: 13, 14 |
| 6.3.b | Re-direct priorities based on assessment findings. | P | P | MPT: 13, 14 |

# Area 7 Transportation

## GENERAL COMPETENCY 7.1 PREPARE AMBULANCE FOR SERVICE.

| | | PCP | ACP | Reference: Chapters |
|---|---|:---:|:---:|---|
| 7.1a | Conduct vehicle maintenance and safety check. | P | P | MPT: 49 |
| 7.1.b | Recognize conditions requiring removal of vehicle from service. | A | A | MPT: 49 |
| 7.1.c | Utilize all vehicle equipment and vehicle devices within ambulance. | S | S | MPT: 49 |

## GENERAL COMPETENCY 7.2
## DRIVE AMBULANCE OR SIMILAR TYPE VEHICLE.

| | | | | |
|---|---|:---:|:---:|---|
| 7.2.a | Utilize defensive driving techniques. | A | A | MPT: 49 |
| 7.2.b | Utilize safe emergency driving techniques. | A | A | MPT: 49 |
| 7.2.c | Drive in a manner that ensures patient comfort and a safe environment for all passengers. | A | A | MPT: 49 |

## GENERAL COMPETENCY 7.3
## TRANSFER PATIENT TO AIR AMBULANCE.

| | | | | |
|---|---|:---:|:---:|---|
| 7.3.a | Create safe landing zone for rotary-wing aircraft. | A | A | MPT: 49 |
| 7.3.b | Safely approach stationary rotary-wing aircraft. | A | A | MPT: 49 |
| 7.3.c | Safely approach stationary fixed-wing aircraft. | A | A | MPT: 49 |
| 7.4.a | Prepare patient for air medical transport. | A | A | MPT: 49 |
| 7.4.b | Recognize the stressors of flight on patient, crew, and equipment and the implications for patient care. | A | A | MPT: 49 |

*To see the complete National Occupational Competency Profiles, including the CCP competencies, visit the Paramedic Association of Canada Web site at: www.paramedic.ca.*

# GLOSSARY

**abandonment:** Terminating medical care without legal excuse or turning care over to personnel one knows or ought to know do not have the training and expertise appropriate for the medical need of the patient.

**Advanced Care Paramedic (ACP):** A qualified Primary Care Paramedic who has successfully completed an Advanced Care Paramedic training program in accordance with the Canadian National Occupational Competency Profiles (NOCP) and approved by the province or territory. The ACP must also be authorized by a medical director to perform controlled acts.

**Advanced Life Support (ALS):** The provision of care that paramedics or allied healthcare professionals render, including advanced airway management, defibrillation, intravenous therapy, and medication administration.

**assault:** The intentional threat of or application of physical force against another person without legal justification.

**attending paramedic:** Sometimes referred to as the "lead paramedic"; the person, on a particular call, who has taken responsibility for the overall management of the call and the patient. The attending paramedic will assume a lead role at the scene and will be the one to attend to the patient en route to the hospital. Paramedics generally work in pairs, alternating the roles of attending paramedic and driver paramedic.

**automated external defibrillator (AED):** A device used in cardiac arrest to perform a computer analysis of the patient's cardiac rhythm and to deliver defibrillatory shocks when indicated.

**automatic vehicle location (AVL):** A radio communications subsystem that uses one or more electronic methods periodically to determine the position of a land, marine, or air vehicle and to relay that information by radio to a communications centre.

**basic life support (BLS):** Care provided by individuals trained in first aid, cardiopulmonary resuscitation, and other noninvasive care.

**client:** Note that the word "client" and "patient" are used interchangeably.

**continuous quality improvement:** A management approach to customer service and organizational performance that includes constant monitoring, evaluation, decisions, appropriate corrective actions, and re-evaluation.

**controlled medical act:** Also referred to as simply "controlled act"; a procedure that has a high element of risk if not done correctly and by a competent person and is therefore restricted by law to physicians or trained professionals operating under medical directives. These acts include, for example, communicating a diagnosis, giving injections, and using electricity or certain forms of energy to treat a patient.

**cultural competence:** A group of skills, attitudes, and knowledge that allows a paramedic to work effectively and with sensitivity with diverse racial, ethnic, and social groups.

**differential diagnosis:** A short list of possible causes of the patient's complaint.

**emergency medical services (EMS):** A national network of services coordinated to provide aid and medical assistance from primary response to definitive care; it involves personnel trained in rescue, stabilization, transport, and advanced management of traumatic and medical emergencies.

**emergency medical technician:** A person who has completed training based on the EMT or EMT–Paramedic National Standard Curriculum. The EMT training is a BLS level of training, while the EMT-P training is similar to Canada's Advanced Care Paramedic (ACP) training and includes advanced training in patient assessment, cardiac rhythm interpretation, defibrillation, drug therapy, and advanced airway management.

**express consent:** Explicit consent in words (oral or written).

**first responder:** One who, in the early stages of an incident, is responsible for the preservation of life and the provision of patient care. A first responder may be a bystander trained in first aid, a firefighter, or a medically trained paramedic. First responders, by definition, do not transport patients to the hospital but provide care until an ambulance arrives.

**forcible confinement:** Unlawfully confining, imprisoning, or holding another person against his or her will.

**hemodynamic monitoring device:** A device that measures the pressure exerted by blood against the wall of a blood vessel (artery or vein) or a chamber of the heart. Paramedics use that measurement to help determine how well organs, particularly the brain, are perfused. Primary and Advanced Care Paramedics typically use simple noninvasive hemodynamic monitoring devices such as a manual or automatic blood pressure cuff. Critical Care Paramedics also use invasive hemodynamic devices that measure pressure directly from within an artery, a large vein, or the heart. This provides more accurate and continuous monitoring.

**history of the presenting illness or injury (HPI):** A chronological description of the development of the patient's present illness or of events leading up to an injury.

**hospital diversion:** A policy or procedure, usually created through agreements among ambulance services, local hospitals, a medical director, and the communications centre, to allow paramedics to bypass the closest hospital to go to the next closest hospital when the ER at the closest one is overcrowded.

**implied consent:** Consent implied by the circumstances or conduct of the patient, which may include a presumption that an unconscious or incompetent person would consent to life-saving care.

**incident management system (IMS):** System used for the management of multiple casualty incidents involving responsibility for command, designation, and coordination of triage, treatment, transport, and staging; sometimes called *incident command system.*

**informed consent:** Consent obtained after disclosure of pertinent information, including the material or probable risks of receiving or refusing treatment.

**injury risk:** Real or potential hazards that put individuals at increased risk for sustaining an injury.

**injury surveillance:** The ongoing systematic collection, analysis, and interpretation of injury data essential to the planning, implementation, and evaluation of public health practice.

**involuntary consent:** Consent that is granted by authority of law.

**mass casualty incident (MCI):** An event for which available resources are insufficient to manage the number of casualties.

**mechanical ventilator:** A mechanical device designed to deliver air into the lungs, under pressure, at a rate and volume controlled by the operator.

**medical directive:** A written statement by the medical director that describes a medical condition and the treatment to be rendered. A medical directive can be a standing order or a simple instruction to contact a physician for direction under certain circumstances. It may include protocols for medical acts, as well as policies and procedures for tasks that are not medically defined, such as determining a hospital destination.

**negligence:** An act or omission that fails to meet the standard of care reasonably expected of a prudent paramedic with appropriate training, having regard to all of the circumstances.

**out-of-hospital care:** Broadly speaking, care provided for patients who may or may not be transported to the hospital.

**prehospital:** Medical treatment in the field before transport and transfer of care to a medical facility. This term presumes the patient will be transported to a hospital.

**Primary Care Paramedic (PCP):** A qualified person who has successfully completed a Primary Care Paramedic training program in accordance with the Canadian National Occupational Competency Profiles (NOCP) and approved by the province or territory. The PCP must also be authorized by a medical director to perform a limited number of controlled acts.

**primary injury prevention:** The practice of preventing an injury from occurring.

**primary problem:** The underlying problem or most probable cause of the patient's signs and symptoms.

**provisional diagnosis or field diagnosis:** A tentative diagnosis based on clinical findings and a high degree of probability. In the absence of laboratory test results, a provisional diagnosis may be the basis for initiating immediate treatment to avoid harm.

**reciprocity:** The practice of granting an individual licensure, certification, or registration based on licensure, certification, or registration by another province or territory.

**scope of practice:** A range of skills (controlled acts) that paramedics are allowed and expected to perform when indicated.

**secondary injury prevention:** The practice of preventing injury at the event phase. This may include promoting the use of protective gear or designing objects to incorporate injury-prevention features (e.g., air bags in cars).

**standards of practice:** A body of knowledge or benchmarks for conduct and performance of duties applicable to an individual with the training and experience of a paramedic; an example is The National Occupational Competency Profiles (NOCP).

**standing order:** Specific treatment protocols that can be used by paramedics in the absence of online (direct) medical direction when delay in treatment would harm the patient or when the treatment is considered reasonable and safe.

**tertiary injury prevention:** The practice of preventing injury in the postevent phase; for example, cooling and protecting a burn to prevent deeper burning and reduce the risk of subsequent infection.

**triage bypass:** A medical directive allowing a paramedic crew, with approval from the emergency medical dispatcher, to bypass the closest hospital so that the patient can be transported to a hospital providing specialized care.

**triage nurse:** A nurse in the ER who takes the initial report from the paramedic and is responsible for sorting and categorizing patients according to severity of illness or injury.

# INDEX

Note: Page numbers followed by "f" indicate figures; "t" tables; "b" boxes.